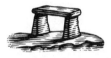

rockbench

PUBLISHING

courageous thought leadership content

PJoe
Public
DOESN'T
CARE
Yabout
Your
HOSPITAL

(*A Manifesto for Transforming Healthcare Marketing*)

CHRIS BEVOLO

RockBench Publishing Corp.
6101 Stillmeadow Dr., Nashville, TN 37211
www.rockbench.com

Printed in the United States of America
First Edition 2011

Published simultaneously in electronic format

Library of Congress Control Number: 2011933659

ISBN: 9781605440101

Table of Contents

Acknowledgements

This is a book I've dreamed of writing and there are many people to thank for making the dream a reality.

First, to all those who contributed to the book with insights, quotes, opinions and push back, thank you. I've always believed dialogue is one of the best ways to learn, and I learned a lot in the writing of this book. There were also a lot of people whose thoughts I'd love to have included in this book – we'll get you in next time. I'd also like to extend my gratitude to all my clients, associates, vendors, partners, prospects and competitors: Your stories and experiences have shaped my views over the years, and this book would not have been possible without the trials, tribulations and triumphs you have had in this crazy world of healthcare marketing.

A heartfelt thanks also goes to the team at Interval, for their support of my "writing black holes" in iCal and for inspiring many of the thoughts and concepts found in this book. Special thanks to Adam Meyer, our creative director, who has always pushed me to think about new things, embrace new ways, and stretch my marketing brain.

To David Baker, my long-trusted consultant and Sherpa, thanks for providing the opportunity to publish this book through RockBench Publishing. To Gienna Shaw, who gave me my first (and second) opportunities to publish a book. And thanks also to

Helena Bouchez, who provided encouragement and "tell it like it is" feedback over the long slog toward the completion of this journey.

Finally, I'd like to thank my kids, Jack, Julia and Callie, who endured approximately 700 instances of "hold on, just a minute" as I typed a thought or corrected a passage. I hope the investment I've made in writing this book will inspire you to make the most of your life as you grow older. Thanks also to my parents for their lifelong support. And to Tonya – thanks for being there with me for the duration. I love you all.

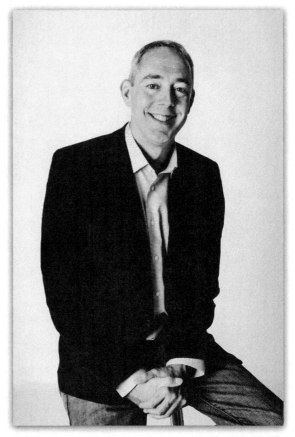

Author, Chris Bevolo

ChrisBevolo.com

About the Author

Chris Bevolo is a healthcare marketing change agent. His mission: Inspire, persuade and support hospital and health system leaders to evolve their approach to healthcare marketing.

A nationally recognized futurist, author and speaker on healthcare marketing, strategy and branding, Chris helps organizations to better understand key trends in healthcare competition, branding and consumerism. He then helps marketing leaders create strategies that will effectively leverage those trends. He is best known, however, for helping healthcare organizations re-envision what their marketing could be, re-energizing management and inspiring staff to think bigger and act differently.

As an educator and bridge builder, Chris not only helps healthcare marketing executives build and strengthen communications with top leadership and key influencers, he also assists with practical advice and support on specific healthcare marketing challenges.

Chris is a frequent keynote speaker and featured presenter at national healthcare conferences on the topics of marketing, branding, innovation, the patient experience, and consumer trends. He is the author of two previous books, "A Marketer's Guide to Measuring Results" (2010) and "A Marketer's Guide to Brand Strategy" (HealthLeaders Media, 2008), as well as numerous articles and papers on healthcare marketing and branding. Chris earned an M.B.A. at the University of St. Thomas in Minneapolis and holds a B.S. in journalism and mass communication from Iowa State University.

As president and founder of the Minneapolis-based healthcare marketing agency Interval (est. 1995 as Geiger Bevolo), Chris and his team have put the concepts outlined in this book into practice many times. They've developed successful marketing campaigns, brand strategies, patient experience innovation and more for healthcare organizations such as Inova Health System, Children's Hospitals and Clinics of Minnesota, Allegiance Health, St. Joseph's Hospital, Woodwinds Health Campus, North Memorial Health Care, Hudson Hospital, Blue Cross and Blue Shield of Minnesota, Brookings Health System, LifeSource, and the Minnesota Hospital Association.

INTRODUCTION:
Current state

A couple of years ago, I worked with a small clinical group to develop a brand strategy and identity for a new clinic they were planning. The focus of the clinic was a tiny subsegment of cardiac patients. So tiny that only three systems in the state offered a program directed at the affliction. New patient goals were to be measured in the dozens. We kicked off our process with a cross-functional meeting, with key physicians, operational managers, nurses and care coordinators in attendance. Given our very targeted audience, I made an explicit attempt to manage expectations regarding brand building and marketing. At one point in the kick-off meeting, I off-handedly joked: "At least we don't have to worry about billboards this time." Laughs all around, and the meeting proceeded apace.

A week later, the group reconvened to further discuss key components of their brand strategy. The meeting was going along fine until, inevitably, inescapably, inexorably, it happened. Apropos of virtually nothing, one of the cardiologists spoke up:

"I know we dismissed the idea of billboards last time," he said. "But I've been thinking more about it. I know our audience is really small, but maybe there's an intersection in town where the traffic patterns are just right, one that might make a billboard a smart option."

As the sun rises in the east, and the tax man comes in April, so too does the doctor request a billboard. And so goes the current state of healthcare marketing. But it doesn't have to be this way...

This book is a call to arms. A battle cry to healthcare marketers near and far to rise up and lead our organizations to better futures through better marketing. This manifesto – based on five core changes – can serve as our guide and rallying point for shaking off the outdated and ineffective methods of the past, and embracing a mindset to lead us into the future. For some of you, the ideas in this book may be old hat. You, then, are the front line in this revolution, the leaders of our movement. For many of you – marketing and organizational leaders alike – this book will contain concepts that at best may feel foreign, at worst like blasphemy. But there's nothing wrong with dissent and debate – a healthy dialogue will only help move us forward. At the very least, I hope this book will drive that dialogue. At best, I hope marketing leaders in hospitals, health systems, physician groups and other providers will adopt these philosophies and use them to boldly usher our industry into an age of marketing enlightenment. So, let us begin.

The past as prologue

There are a number of key reasons why transformation of healthcare marketing is an urgent necessity. To understand the situation today, it helps to review how history brought us to this point. Why, as an industry, do we struggle with marketing our organizations? Why are we behind most all other industries – including healthcare sectors such as pharma or med-tech – in understanding and valuing marketing? How did we get here?

In a nutshell, it's because of the relatively "recent" need for hospitals and health systems to *compete for business*. Up until the 1980's, the need for competitive strategies – and thus marketing – often just wasn't necessary. Here's how I described the phenomenon in "A Marketer's Guide to Brand Strategy":

"Until the 1970s, 'competition' was not on the strategic radar for most healthcare providers. With a few exceptions, healthcare providers adhered to ideology expressed by Sir William Osler, 'The practice of medicine is an art, not a trade; a calling, not a business.' This mindset began to change after the HMO Act of 1973, though real market pressures didn't begin to hit until the 1980's with the advent of managed

care. Suddenly, patient flow was restricted, and healthcare providers had to consider ways to keep patient volumes up. Most hospitals and health systems didn't even have marketing departments until the 1980's. During the 1980's and 1990's, many healthcare organizations grew in size and scope, many large national chains were created (such as Humana and HCA) and physician-owned hospitals and specialty clinics became more prominent. All of this ushered in a new, highly competitive atmosphere."[1]

That means the industry as a whole is still relatively low on the learning curve when it comes to leveraging marketing to gain competitive advantage. One result of this history is a class of healthcare leadership that is, in general, behind when it comes to marketing. In so many cases, marketing and branding are simply not understood – or worse, not valued – by those who lead our organizations. No matter how smart or creative the marketing department is, how sophisticated the strategy, how clever the campaign, if the CEO or the head surgeon doesn't get it, it won't fly. Take this experience, for example:

I once worked with a senior marketing executive at a health system who was talking with her CEO about the need to prioritize the organization's consumer marketing efforts. There were far too many service line initiatives on the table, and the marketer was concerned about the level of commitment needed to properly promote all the targeted service lines. In addition, argued the marketer, we can't expect consumers to remember and prioritize our organization around so many service lines because consumers can really only handle a few key messages or differentiation points. The argument was based on the classic principles of *positioning*, which states that because consumers are overwhelmed with inputs from the market, they slot products and services in a way that allows them to retain and value only a few offerings in each segment (positioning is described in more detail in Chapter 1). In this case, the marketer hadn't thought to lay out the argument for positioning – why would she? Wasn't it understood? Yet the CEO stopped her short and said, "Well, how do we know that consumers can't absorb all of these messages? I think you need to pull together some research and build a case for that. I'm not sure I'm convinced."

The marketer was flummoxed. How in the world would she "prove" the idea of positioning – a basic business principle upon which many other marketing beliefs and philosophies are built? If someone came to you and said "I'm not certain the earth isn't flat – could you build a case to prove that?" Where would you begin? Of course the earth isn't flat – that was proved centuries ago and we've all moved on.

In their defense, many of these leaders don't have formal marketing education or experience. But in its absence, instead of trusting their marketing leaders, they fall back on what they've seen before or what they currently see in the healthcare market. Because both of these sources all too often reflect bad or "old school" marketing, the cycle repeats itself. There can also be political pressure internally to "make the physicians happy," which often means giving in to the demand for wrong-headed marketing tactics like promoting gallbladder surgery using billboards and newspaper advertising. So often I hear from our clients, "Yes, we know it's not effective, but do it anyway. It will make them happy."

But it's not just leadership that needs help with marketing. The same could be said of the other power players in a hospital or health system – physicians, service line directors, operational managers and other C-suiters. These influencers also rarely have marketing experience, leading to a reinforcement of bad strategies and old tactics. Finally, in many cases, those responsible for healthcare marketing struggle *themselves* to fully understand or leverage marketing as a discipline. Many healthcare marketers have education or experience in communications and public relations, or some other related discipline. Some have no formal marketing education and many absorb marketing responsibilities after starting out in other departments such as HR, operations, or even clinical. (If that describes you, don't worry. This book will help crystallize and prioritize the critical philosophies and strategies you need to follow.)

The times, they are a changin'

As if operating in an industry that is still playing catch up with the rest of the business world when it comes to marketing is not hard enough, consider that over the past several years, a number of trends have collided to produce a new dynamic that we are only just now beginning to feel. At the core of this dynamic is the "empowered consumer."

There are three core elements driving this major sea-change. The first is consumer *choice*. In his famed book "The World Is Flat," Thomas Friedman leads off his treatise by using the example of overseas "nighthawk" radiology services to help illustrate his contention that geographic barriers to trade are crumbling.[2] Medical tourism is a growing business, but it's no longer restricted to international destinations. Recently, home improvement mammoth Lowe's announced a program to send its employees from all over the country to the Cleveland Clinic to receive heart care, signaling the power of "domestic" medical tourism.[3] In addition, telemedicine is allowing home-based diagnoses and treatments that were unthinkable 20 years ago. Then consider all the new entrants into the market that compete with traditional providers of healthcare, such as the mini-clinics found in Wal-Mart and CVS pharmacy locations around the U.S., or the diabetes coaching service recently launched by Walgreens.[4] These market forces and more combine to give healthcare consumers more choices than ever before.

Second, consumers have access to more healthcare *information* than ever before. The Internet has enabled consumer choice by allowing consumers to search through volumes of information on available healthcare options. Seemingly every week, a new web-based resource is launched that rates physicians and hospitals in the areas of quality, price, experience or more, often containing a plethora of reviews from current and former patients. In fact, consumers and patients alike are driving much of the discussion on healthcare, whether through formal health forums like the website PatientsLikeMe.com, or through feedback on newspaper comment boards, Twitter and Facebook. Search engines bring dozens of choices to our fingertips in an instant, and mobile technology is allowing us to find what we want, wherever we are.

Finally, consider the fuel on the fire: *money.* More consumers are facing increased out-of-pocket costs, thanks to HSAs, HRAs and other high-deductible plans. As consumers spend more of their own money for care, they are beginning to search for and value factors applied in other purchasing decisions – convenience, quality, service, and price. It's one thing to pay a $10 copay to see a specialist and incur a slew of tests – it's another to have to foot the bill for such an encounter, which could run into the thousands of dollars. The change in thinking is inevitable: Do I really need this treatment? Why does it cost so much? Is there a more convenient way to access this service? *What are my other options?*

Of course, many of the traditional drivers of consumer choice in healthcare – physician referral, insurance coverage and proximity – still play a vital role in influencing which patients go to which doctor, hospital or health system. There is no doubt, however, that the trends above are impacting our organizations, as are generational shifts in how people choose care. (Generally speaking, the older you are, the more likely you are to follow your doctor's recommendation blindly, while the younger you are, the more likely you are to guide your own care decisions.) You may certainly question how much the empowered consumer really has made an impact to date. But consider the following blog post I wrote in the spring of 2009 on the economic crisis and its effect on how consumers make healthcare decisions (especially given that the post was written at the beginning of what is still a very difficult economic situation in the U.S.). Arguably, the crisis has eased in some ways, but the behaviors triggered by that event persist and in fact are becoming even more prevalent. Here it is again, in its entirety:

The economic crisis: Tipping point for healthcare consumer behavior?

With their own money on the line, consumers are beginning to use the same value criteria for healthcare decisions – service, price, experience, brand equity and more – as they do with other purchasing decisions. To date, however, the new healthcare "consumerism" has not led to a widespread change in consumer behavior. But this nation's current economic crisis may well be the tipping point; the driver of fundamental change in how and when consumers engage hospitals and health systems.

The Tide is Turning

In 2007, roughly 10% of those with health insurance had some form of consumer-driven coverage, defined as an HRA, HSA or other high-deductible option. Combined with the uninsured, adult U.S. consumers with significant skin in the game are still in the minority. But given the accelerated adoption of consumer-driven plans and the current economic crisis, dramatic change is coming.

Many predict adoption of consumer-driven plans will rise to 15% in 2009. According to Clayton Christensen, author of "The Innovator's Prescription: A Disruptive Solution for Health Care," that adoption will likely hit 50% by 2013, and 90% by 2016.[5] (His book "The Innovator's Dilemma," cites research that shows the rate of adoption of innovation typically starts slow, then hits a tipping point when widespread use skyrockets.)

Tough financial times are causing more employers to drop health insurance altogether. A new survey by Hewitt Associates shows that 19% of employers are planning to stop offering health benefits over the next three to five years, a response nearly five times higher than the previous year.[6]

The economic crisis has led to growing unemployment (8% nationally at this writing). Many expect that number to reach 10% before the end of 2009. This restructuring of the national economy is ratcheting up the number of uninsured and underinsured.

Even those that have avoided job loss are tightening their belts in significant ways. Not only is income being threatened, but the old fall-back resources of home equity lines and credit cards are drying up. Many are watching every penny as their spending resources dry up, and pulling back on spending "just in case" of job loss, medical emergency or other dire situations.

All of these trends are causing an increase in exposure to out-of-pocket healthcare costs for consumers, and the impact has been significant. According to a recent Kaiser Family Foundation Health Tracking Poll, 53% of respondents said their households had cut back on healthcare in the previous year due to cost concerns.[7] A recent Wall Street Journal online piece noted that retailer CVS is closing 90 MinuteClinics for the season, to "align with consumer demand."[8] Many hospitals and health systems are reporting dramatic drops in utilization. Summing it up recently was David Wessner, CEO of Park Nicollet Health Services in Minneapolis, who was quoted in a recent Minneapolis Star Tribune story on the financial ills of hospitals. Wessner said: "We're seeing that demand is far more elastic than it was in other years."[9]

Of course, much of the drop in healthcare utilization attributed to the economic crisis could be seen as short-term. When the economy recovers, consumers will return to regular healthcare usage, and all will be fine. But chances are many of the changes we're seeing will become permanent.

A permanent shift?

Economic crisis has driven societal behavior change before. For example, those who lived through the Great Depression of the 1930's (often referred to as the "Greatest Generation"), were very cautious with their money. Debt was considered bad, as was spending beyond your means. The norm was to save carefully to buy a home or car, and to have a significant cash reserves at the ready to meet unexpected, emergency expenses such as the need for medical attention. Economic crisis taught this generation (the youngest of which are in their 70's now) the critical importance of making smart financial decisions, of not over-extending themselves, and the value of saving first and spending later. These financially conservative attitudes did not change until the next (Baby Boomer) generation.

10

Will we see the same shift in financial attitudes as a result of this crisis? A recent article in Time talked about how consumers are walking into stores with a new level of negotiating power:

"Store owners will tell you horror stories about shoppers with attitude, who walk in demanding discounts and flaunt their new power at every turn. They wince as they sense bad habits forming: Will people expect discounts forever? Will their hard-won brand luster be forever cheapened, especially for items whose allure depends on their being ridiculously priced?" [10]

Once new consumer habits are formed, it's very difficult to change them. Given how most of us have been blind to the true cost of healthcare our entire lives, it's not surprising that old habits in choosing care die hard. Note the struggles of Carol.com in the Twin Cities market, which had trouble convincing enough consumers to shop for care through their innovative web site. Could the shift of greater out-of-pocket exposure to more and more people trigger a permanent change in healthcare behavior?

The impact on healthcare providers

The economic storm will pass eventually, but what if the newfound priorities of healthcare consumers stick around? The impact would be profound for healthcare providers:

- *The current drop in volumes may be a permanent reduction of utilization, as consumers avoid non-essential treatment, stretch out physician visits, and find lower-cost alternatives (alternative medicine, "homemade" remedies and more). Of course, the wave of Baby Boomers and their increased need for care may cancel this out, or override it altogether.*

- *Price shopping will become the norm, as consumers carefully consider their alternatives and negotiate for lower costs whenever possible.*

- *While price will be one value driver, others such as convenience, experience and service will continue to grow in importance, relative to clinical quality, as patients demand more for their money.*

- *Competition in the healthcare market will become even more intense, while the resources to grow market share, increase volumes and build brands become increasingly scarce.*

The healthcare hurricane is coming

The potential impact of consumer-driven healthcare on providers is like a hurricane forming in the Gulf of Mexico. The storm is out there but no one knows where it will hit: North, South or direct? Will it stay at its current level of strength, fizzle out before reaching shore, or grow to a Category 5 "killer"? Until recently, the "consumer-driven" hurricane was too small and too far out at sea to be a major cause of concern for providers. But depending on what happens with the economy over the next few months, it could rapidly grow in power and race toward shore. Is your hospital or health system ready? [11]

Other contributing factors

What about healthcare reform? As of this writing, the true shape of reform was still being debated, as organizations across the U.S. tried to untangle the complicated guidelines of the Affordable Care Act to understand how best to adapt to the potentially significant changes. But from what I've read and from those I've talked with, healthcare reform will likely continue the trends noted above, if not accelerate them. And at the very least, reform does not change the fundamental concept that provider organizations will need to continue to compete for business. And as long as there is a need for competition, there will be a need for us to conduct effective marketing.

As if healthcare marketers didn't have enough to deal with, two other movements are impacting our industry, and are demanding a better approach from marketers. First, in spring of 2010, a state legislator from Vermont proposed a law that would prohibit hospitals from spending money on advertising or marketing. Democrat Steve Maier didn't approve of that type of spending when the state struggles year after year to contain skyrocketing healthcare costs:

"It's not producing health care," Maier said in an interview in the Burlington Free Press.[12]

Second is the growing trend of hospitals and health systems engaging productivity consultants to investigate and recommend cost savings throughout the organization. Typically, the recommendations are tied to a benchmark of similar organizations throughout the country, so a hospital may find it stands at the 78th percentile in spending on its oncology service line, and then can peg cost cutting to attaining a goal of, say, 50%. These assessments have been around for some time, no doubt. But they seem to have accelerated dramatically in the wake of the Great Recession. And it seems that in almost every case where one of these consultants is brought in, marketing takes a hit, sometimes a significant one, in overall budget allotment. Often, FTEs are reduced as well. In both cases, the need for marketers to deliver effective strategies and results is only accentuated.

An urgent need to change

To put it simply, it's a whole new ballgame, folks. All of these reasons – a late start to marketing as an industry, under-informed leadership, empowered consumers, the Great Recession and extended economic downturn, healthcare reform, delivering more for less – add up to a simple and urgent truth:

Those responsible for marketing hospitals, health systems and other provider organizations must deliver more, demonstrable value from their efforts than ever before.

- We must deliver higher volumes, physician visits, surgeries, diagnostics, market share, referrals, web traffic, social media engagement and more.

- We must increase our results with less budget, and likely, fewer staff members.

- We must be more effective in targeting the right audience at the right time.

- We must build better, more differentiated brands.

- We must respond in the face of unknown or murky regulatory changes.

- We must be sensitive to the ongoing scrutiny of our efforts from government, the media and the public.

- We must do all this in an ever-shifting media landscape.

We must transform how we market our healthcare organizations!

This book is my attempt to prioritize the most important changes necessary to make that transformation happen.

Who can benefit from reading this book?

First and foremost, this book is for all those who serve in marketing, communications and public relations roles at hospitals and health systems in the United States. For that matter, anyone who serves in those roles at any organization that provides healthcare – clinics, specialty centers, mini-clinics, etc. – will benefit from the contents.

But this book is also for anyone in these organizations who asks for, participates in, or approves marketing activities. Typically, that includes organizational leaders – CEOs, COOs, and administrators. It also includes service line directors, operational managers, and of course, physicians. When I speak at healthcare marketing conferences about any of the changes proposed in this book, I'm often preaching to the choir. In many ways, it's more important that organizational leaders, operational leaders and physicians read this book. It is their understanding of the transformational philosophies found here that would allow for the biggest leap forward in improved healthcare marketing.

While it may be obvious, it's also worth noting that this book is for those who understand the need to market hospitals and health systems, and who believe in the value of marketing and branding in healthcare. This book won't dip into a debate about the U.S. health care system, the effectiveness or ineffectiveness of the system, the tension between for-profit and non-profit missions, whether hospitals should be allowed to advertise, the quasi-competitive nature of this industry, or any societal issues related to delivering care in this country. We face a reality – whether we like or not – of a healthcare system that requires and encourages healthcare organizations to compete, and this book is unabashedly about helping healthcare organizations do just that.

A point about verbiage

As I've mentioned, this book is aimed at what I call "provider organizations," or those organizations that provide care to patients at any level. This includes hospitals, health systems, clinics, physician groups, specialty centers, diagnostic centers and mini-clinics. With that in mind, I realize the title, "Joe Public Doesn't Care About Your Hospital," may be misleading. This isn't just about marketing a hospital, it's about marketing any of the organizations noted above, and in most cases, figuring out how to market multiple providers within one healthcare organization. So try not to get too hung up on the word "hospital." As you'll note throughout the book, I often interchange hospital with health system, or use them together to stress a point. In the end, I could have just substituted "provider organization" so that I'm covering all the bases, but I don't believe that resonates as well (i.e. "Joe Public Doesn't Care About Your Provider Organization" just doesn't have that same ring to it). So in most places, you'll see the descriptor "healthcare marketing." As long as we all agree that for the purposes of this book, I'm referring to providers, not other sectors of healthcare (insurers, pharma and med tech), then I think we'll be in good shape.

Also, it has often been pointed out to me that given the prominent role of women in making healthcare decisions, I should refer to Joe Public as a she, not a he. Granted, women are typically the primary audience for healthcare marketers, and perhaps rightly so. But the clichéd metaphor I'm using here for illustrative purposes, is, in fact, *Joe Public*. Switching to Josephine Public or Jody Public just doesn't have the same punch. So, for clarity's sake, please assume that whenever I mention Joe Public by name or as a "he," I intend that reference to be gender neutral.

Five changes for healthcare marketing

The five changes for transforming healthcare marketing outlined here are based on my 12 years of experience working in this industry, and while some of them address obvious issues or challenges in this industry, I still experience the need to revisit them on an almost daily basis. For each, I've tried to provide a clear description of the problem at hand, a compelling argument for why change is needed, and suggestions for how you can affect appropriate change. I've even provided a satirical opening to each chapter using grist from the Weekly Probe, my agency's version of The Onion for healthcare marketing, to help set the stage. (For a fun 20 minutes of humorous takes on our beloved industry, check out www.weeklyprobe.com.) My hope is that I provide so much ammunition in each chapter that you and your peers will be inspired to rise up, embrace and implement the changes at hand.

Following is a brief overview of the five suggested changes, followed by some perspective on how to qualify them.

Visit WeeklyProbe.com

Change One: Joe Public doesn't care about your hospital

One of the greatest errors of healthcare marketing is the assumption that consumer audiences care about your organization as much as you do. This sin is repeated over and over, in organization after organization, and the prevalence of this problem (and the resulting ineffectiveness) is the reason the book is titled after this change. Without the ability to move past this road block, it will be impossible for healthcare organizations to fully embrace the other changes.

Change Two: Out with the old, in with the new

This chapter speaks to the need for healthcare marketers to move beyond traditional methods that are no longer as effective; methods that, unfortunately, are very commonplace in our field. It conveys the attitude you'll need to adopt if you want to break ties with the past and move into a brighter, and more successful, future.

Change Three: Breaking bad habits

Throughout our industry, many of us are guilty of falling into habits which hamstring our ability to deliver successful marketing. For example, driving healthcare marketing strategies based on internal pressures ("politically driven" marketing) or always following what others are doing in the market rather than setting our own course ("Me-too" marketing). Becoming aware of and then consciously replacing unproductive habits with those proven more effective will help us to become much more effective marketers.

Change Four: Breathing life into zombie brands

Most healthcare leaders have a hard time understanding the definition of branding, let alone working to build their organization's brand in a strategic way. "Zombie brands" are brands that are left to wander the market without guidance or support from their own organizations, and they must be replaced by brands that are actively defined, developed and managed.

Change Five: Measure, measure, measure

Once we've convinced leadership to let us work in a new way, we must prove our new approaches to healthcare marketing are actually working. That means we must put into place the structure that will allow us to measure the results of our efforts. From a career-perspective, healthcare marketers should consider marketing measurement a "life or death" proposition.

There are undoubtedly many other ways healthcare marketing could change for the better, and some may be more fundamental or profound than the five listed here. But I believe that the adoption of these five core philosophies together can transform healthcare marketing. These particular changes were selected not just because of their "truthiness" (hat tip to Stephen Colbert), but also because of the great need I saw in defining them and spreading the word about them. When made in concert, I believe these five changes have the greatest potential to help healthcare organizations move forward and embrace new and better ways to connect with consumers.

The ideas you will find here are based primarily on my experiences over the past 12 years in healthcare marketing, the observations I and others in my firm have made, and discussions I've had with others I know and trust in the industry. My goal was not to create a scientific case but rather to continue the conversation that was started on my blog and in conference rooms, between colleagues and clients and the media. There is plenty of room for debate and controversy. In publishing this book, I am issuing a standing invitation to join what I hope is a lively and illuminating conversation. At the very least, you will better understand the issues at hand and broaden your perspectives on them. At best, as an industry, we can come to a consensus on some or all of the ideas and move our discipline forward in amazing ways.

So, are you ready? Let's dig into the five changes I believe will transform healthcare marketing and get this party started.

CHAPTER ONE:

Joe Public doesn't care about your hospital

From the WeeklyProbe:

Ad kudos of the week: Embracing narcissism

At Circle J Medical Center, they are committed disciples of the old marketing axiom, "What's in it for me?"

"Every day we ask ourselves, in what new way can we talk about ourselves, call attention to ourselves, shine the spotlight on ourselves?" says senior market director Joseph Kool. "Truly, what is in it for us?"

The latest incarnation of the organization's marketing strategy is a new ad campaign featuring their own doctors and touting the organization's penchant for winning awards, hiring attractive staff and its overall awesomeness. The campaign has an internal component as well, featuring mirrors hung at ten-foot increments throughout the hallways so staff can admire themselves as they pass by.

"What makes this campaign so successful, other than the fact that we rock, is its uniqueness," says Kool. "As far as we know, not many other hospitals are talking about themselves in their advertising, so our message is bound to stand out and really resonate with customers."

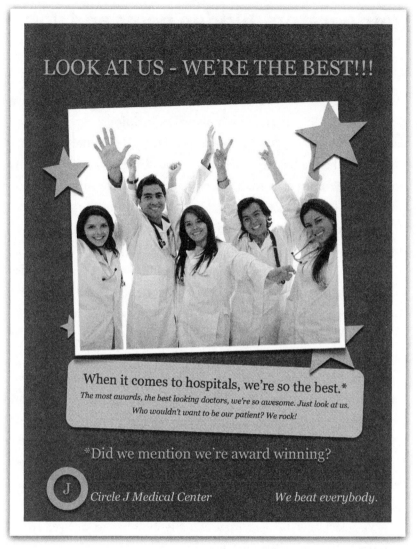

Advertisement featured on WeeklyProbe.com

Refrigerators, hidden gems and you

This is the first chapter in the book for a number of reasons. First, it makes for a great book title. Second, it is perhaps the most frustrating challenge I run across in my work in healthcare marketing because it is so obvious in its insidiousness and it's so darn pervasive. But perhaps most importantly, I feel like if we can't make this change happen, the rest of the changes outlined in this book will be muted in their effectiveness or worse, impossible to implement.

So, to get things started, let's talk about refrigerators. (I promise there is a healthcare marketing related point to this – bear with me.) First, can you list the top selling refrigerator brands? OK, that's a pretty easy one. I'll bet you got a few. What about the top selling models? Or, what are the different types of refrigerators available? Which manufacturer is known for making the best of each type of refrigerator? Which refrigerator model or brand is rated the highest by *Consumer Reports*? Which brand is known for having the most cutting-edge refrigeration technology? What, by the way, *are* the latest cutting edge refrigeration technologies? At what price points will you find refrigerators? Who makes the highest-priced refrigerators, and who is known for offering the best value in refrigerators? What colors are available? Finishings? Ice-making functionality? Produce drawer innovations?

A select few readers may actually be able to answer some of these questions. Perhaps they just moved into a new home, or renovated their old one, and had to shop around for a new refrigerator. Perhaps their trusty icebox finally quit working after all these years, and it was time for a replacement. But 95% of us don't know anything about refrigerators because we don't need a refrigerator, and we haven't had to shop for one for years (if ever). And because we don't need one, we don't know much about them, because we don't take time to learn about them. Basically, we don't *care* about them.

And there, ladies and gentlemen, using refrigerators as our analogy, lies the certain but painful truth: because the majority of consumers don't need a hospital, physician or health system at any given time, they don't *care* about those services. They don't *care* that your physicians are board certified. They don't *care* that you were named a top hospital. They don't *care* about your new construction. They don't *care* that you've added a new anesthesiologist. They don't *care* that you have the best people, or the latest technology, or the best amenities. They don't *care* that you care. They just don't flippin' care!!

As the exclamation points belie, I exaggerate to make a point. But only *slightly*. It's natural for an organization to want to promote what makes it great – its award-winning care, its new surgical technology or the new cardiologist on the team. The problem is, most consumers only pay attention to what is relevant to them, or the "What's in it for me?" Certainly, relevant messages aimed at targeted healthcare audiences can be very effective. (For example, orthopedic efforts that target those with demographic attributes that make them likely candidates for a joint pain seminar.) But for those without a current medical issue, health*care* isn't relevant. Even worse, not only is healthcare typically not relevant on any given day, Joe Public doesn't even want to think about medical care (more on that in a bit). And the implications for accepting that Joe Public doesn't care about your hospital can be profound.

The root cause: The hidden gem syndrome

For many of the key influencers in healthcare marketing – executives, physicians, staff, management – there is a prevailing assumption that those in the community really do care about who you are and what your organization has to offer. We call it the Hidden Gem Syndrome, as in "Our hospital is a hidden gem." You probably hear it all the time:

- "If people only knew what great services we offered, we would be set."

- "We're the best kept secret – we need to tell people our story."

- "If we just communicated the quality/scope of our offerings, we'd have all the patients we could handle."

The Hidden Gem Syndrome really is based on three primary misconceptions about your consumer audience:

1. That consumers aren't aware of your offerings (which may or may not be true).

2. That consumers could know, understand, and value all of your offerings (They can't. Consider that according to Clayton Christensen in the "Innovator's Prescription," the average tertiary care academic medical center manages over 100 pathways of care.[13] Do we really expect consumers to be aware of – let alone understand or value – all of those?)

3. That if consumers could know about your offerings, it would be enough to convince people to use your organization. (It's not enough, not by a long shot.)

In essence, the Hidden Gem Syndrome relies on the silver bullet of *awareness*. Simply make people aware of X, Y or Z (or X, Y *and* Z), and they will come running. Of course, those who are pinning the financial survival of a clinic, service line, or hospital on simply "telling their story" are in for a rude awakening. In today's world, marketing starts with awareness, but it ends with compelling customers to choose you over your competitors.

But pinning your hopes on making your consumers aware is flawed for a more fundamental reason – it assumes your consumers actually care about what you have to say. And as I've pointed out, Joe Public doesn't care!

Exactly who is Joe Public?

To understand the potential impact of my contention that Joe Public Doesn't Care About Your Hospital, it helps to clearly define what I mean by Joe Public. First the good news. There are many people in your community who care – and care deeply – about your organization. Consider:

- patients

- patients-to-be

- physicians

- payers

- media

- suppliers

- your board

For various reasons, each of these groups does care about who you are, what your clinical offerings are, what you have to say, and why you're a better choice for their medical needs. But let's look at the two consumer audiences on this list. First, your patients. This is perhaps the most important audience to engage, as they have already used your services. After all, according to conventional wisdom, it costs at least five times as much money to woo a new customer as it does to keep a current one. (Or seven times, or ten times, depending on your version of conventional wisdom.) The great thing about your current patients is that you have an opportunity to ensure loyalty by impressing them with the actual experience you deliver: clinical excellence, amazing customer service, fantastic amenities. This is the most powerful way to build future utilization with consumers – actually impress them with the service you deliver. (See Chapter 4 for more on this concept.) In addition, you know who these people are and what their clinical profile is. Keeping HIPAA in mind, you should be able to communicate with this audience far more effectively than with any other consumer audience.

The next group are patients-to-be, or what could be called prospects. This is the portion of the non-patient population that *does* care about you, because they are in the market for healthcare. They will care about what options they have in the market, which organization has the best physicians, which services are covered by insurance, which facility is closest, etc. They will care about *you* and what you have to say. The problem is, most consumers don't fit into the prospect category, because most consumers aren't looking for healthcare offerings at any given time. Those consumers who aren't patients or prospective patients are the group I call Joe Public. And that group is probably larger than you think.

Counting Joe Public

In 2008, the Center For Studying Health System Change released the results of their latest consumer healthcare survey (the latest version of the study to date). In it, they highlighted the following results related to when consumers engage with healthcare providers:

30

On average, 11% of adults sought a new primary care physician in a given year.

There are any number of reasons someone might seek out a new primary care physician. The most obvious is a move to a new community. But consumers may also lose health insurance coverage because of a change in their existing plan, or as a result of taking a new job – and be forced to find a new doctor. Perhaps a physician has retired, or, in rare cases, has screwed up so badly or has such terrible bedside manner, that a patient must move on. But in our experience – and most would agree – it's pretty rare for people to switch their primary care physician. Other than in the circumstances noted above, once someone starts to see a primary care physician, they tend to stay with that physician. So while the percentage of adults seeing a new primary care physician may change slightly from community to community or from situation to situation, the 11% level seems to make intuitive sense.

On average, 28% of adults sought a new specialist in a given year.

This number is higher because a consumer may need a variety of specialists, but will only have one primary care physician. So, a 50-year-old man moving from Cleveland to Chattanooga may need to find a new cardiologist, endocrinologist and orthopedist. This number is also likely higher because while most people pick one primary care physician and stick with that doctor over the years, they are diagnosed with different ailments over time, requiring the occasional search for a new specialist. And of course, insurance changes, retirement or a bad experience also could drive a change in specialists.

16% of adults sought a medical procedure at a new facility in a given year.

Again, many studies have shown that once people have a clinical encounter with a hospital or health system, they are likely to stay with that organization, unless circumstances force a switch (insurance, moving), or they have a bad experience.

What's the significance of this study? First, we need to take the results with a slight grain of salt, given that they're based on consumer opinions, not on a record of their actual behavior (see Chapter 3 for more on that). But when I run these numbers by those in healthcare, most agree they are a fair representation of consumer activity. The key, then, is that each of these statistics represent consumers seeking a *new* clinical offering. Like home remodelers and movers who are in the rare position of needing to acquire a new refrigerator, these consumers are in the relatively rare position of needing to acquire new care. You may be saying, hey, the figures above add up to more than half the population, what's wrong with that? But we can't take the numbers as a whole, because they undoubtedly reflect the same respondents across the different categories. The person who said they sought out a new facility for a medical procedure due to a move would also have likely answered that they needed a new primary care physician and specialist. Instead of adding these figures together, it's probably best that we average them. Or, using a nice round number, say roughly 25% of people in your market need a new doctor or hospital in a given year (we're not talking about your patients here – of course you're talking to them, right?). That means, conversely, that 75% of people *don't* need a new doctor or hospital. And if 75% of consumers *aren't* in the market for healthcare, then it follows that 75% of consumers don't care about where they receive healthcare.

Which means, dear reader, that *they don't care about your healthcare organization.*

We can play with these numbers, and they certainly will vary from community to community, from service line to service line. Sometimes the percentage will drop, sometimes it will be higher. The point is, roughly speaking, that in any given year, it's fair to say the segment of consumers who don't immediately need what you're offering – Joe Public – represents the majority of your market.

Now that we know who Joe Public is, let's answer the question: why is it so hard to connect with Joe Public?

Why is it so hard to connect with Joe Public?

Let's start with the idea that as a consumer, Joe is under assault. In their groundbreaking *Advertising Age* marketing article, "The Positioning Era Cometh" (1972), brand gurus Al Ries and Jack Trout laid the foundation for modern marketing thinking. Their concept – positioning – was based on the idea that consumers are bombarded with thousands of messages every day, from hundreds of business categories and industries and thousands of products and services. There's no way to process it all, so consumers subconsciously filter and prioritize those that they trust, those that are familiar and those that are relevant.[14]

If positioning was a force in the 1970s, imagine what consumers face today with the advent of the Internet, cable and satellite television, social media, and more. Noted brand expert Marty Neumeier carries the torch for positioning in his 2007 book "Zag," where he advocates that when everyone else zigs, companies should zag (by building true brand differentiation). He supports that point with research that states consumers are hit with more than 3,000 marketing messages per day, yet, according to The American Association of Advertising Agencies research, people are only able to process about 100 messages per day.[15]

As consumers, then, there is no way to process all of the marketing that we're exposed to, so we consciously and unconsciously limit our exposure. How? Consider all the ways in which we select what we want to hear and keep out that which we don't:

- technologies like TiVo and other digital video recorders (DVRs) allow us to skip commercials.

- the existence of satellite radio, iTunes, Pandora and other content provided without advertising.

- the use of RSS feeds and other tools that allow us to sort through all of the information available on the Internet to only bring us what we want to see, cutting out all the rest.

All of these options allow us to avoid commercial communications like never before. The key to breaking through the clutter of thousands of messages and overcoming the hurdles placed in our path by TiVo, iTunes, and more, is to provide messages that are *relevant* to consumers. For most people, the hundreds of auto ads on television fly by with little notice. Until, that is, you are shopping for a car. All of sudden, what was seen before as white noise is suddenly relevant to the viewer. But this is where we get in trouble with Joe Public. As we pointed out earlier, perhaps 50-75% of consumers in any given market have no need to shop for healthcare. My friend and healthcare marketing guru Chris Causey calls healthcare marketing a low-interest category, because nobody thinks about a hospital until they need it. In essence, Joe Public is not buying what we're selling.

Believe it or not, it actually gets worse. Let's go back to the refrigerator example for a moment. If you're not in the market for a new refrigerator, you're unlikely to pay attention to communications from a refrigerator manufacturer. However, it's not like refrigerator ads will offend you or turn you off. Healthcare organizations can't even count on this neutral response. Not only do people not care about hospitals, they actually don't even want to *hear* from them. Who wants to think about a hospital or a doctor if they don't need one? Other than having a baby, there's rarely a positive reason for having to go to a hospital. Hospitals are for the sick and injured, those with chronic diseases, cancer and heart attacks. Yuck – who wants to think about that if they don't have to? In many ways, healthcare organizations are similar to lawyers. Unless you've won the lottery, having to hire a lawyer is typically not a good thing. You're being sued or you're suing. You're fighting over a divorce or a real estate dispute. Whatever it is, it's no fun.

Again, those of us who work in or for healthcare organizations shouldn't take offense at this. If we could keep everyone out of the hospital through some wave of a magic wand, most of us would gladly do so. We are well aware of the amazing medical work that goes on in our organizations – the miracles, really. We know we help thousands of people every day. Hospital and health systems are incredible and critical components of our society. But unfortunately, none of that really helps with Joe Public, or our desire to convince Joe to think of our organization if and when he needs us.

So what are the implications?

If the majority of your consumer audience truly doesn't care about what your healthcare organization has to say, what are the implications for your marketing? For starters, consider the Hidden Gem Syndrome and its tell-tale comments:

- "We're the best kept secret."

- "We're a hidden gem."

- "If we only told people about our service, we would meet our business goals."

Now we can see why simply addressing the Hidden Gem Syndrome doesn't lead to better market share, higher volumes or more visits – *simply telling Joe Public about your services isn't effective because Joe Public doesn't care about your services.* Consider how much of our marketing efforts and resources are oriented toward Joe Public. According to the latest *By the Numbers* publication from the Society For Healthcare Strategy & Market Development (SHSMD), advertising and media expenditures represent one third of the total marketing and communications budget for healthcare organizations.[16] We spend more money trying to connect with Joe Public than any other marketing strategy, yet in most cases, we either are oblivious to or ignore the fact that Joe Public doesn't want to hear from us.

Take for example what happens when a new physician joins our staff. To help promote that physician and build her practice, many organizations run advertisements in the local paper. "Dr. Bevolo has joined our staff as a family practitioner. Call today to make an appointment." But according to the study cited earlier, only 11% of consumers seek out a new primary care physician each year. That means, at best, only 11% of the people who see the ad actually are in the market for a new physician. Or, in more depressing terms, 89% of the readers *aren't*. The point isn't that these ads won't pull in potential new patients – they often do. The point is that as a healthcare marketer, you have a limited budget – most likely, *very* limited. You need to make every marketing dollar count. Given this scenario, is running an ad to promote a new primary care doctor the most effective way to build his or her (and ultimately, your) business?

Here's another example. How many community newsletter articles feature new services, new physicians, new technology, or facility construction updates? Honestly, *who cares?* If you received a newsletter from Whirlpool with information on their latest line of refrigerators, their new fresh fruit technology, a new factory upgrade in Poughkeepsie, and the hiring of their new VP of Human Resources, would you read it?

If Joe Public doesn't care, why oh why do hospitals and health systems spend so much of their valuable marketing dollars promoting all the ratings, rankings and awards they win? For me to be impressed about your award, I have to care about your award. But I don't care about you, so who cares about your award? (Award-based advertising is a common thread throughout this book. I cover it more in depth in Chapter 3.)

Open houses, construction updates, awards, advertising featuring your wonderful staff, awesome physicians or cyber-technology – all of these are chest-pounding, "you"-focused messages that assume the recipient of the message cares about the organization. They don't. So what can you do about it?

Embracing the idea that Joe Public doesn't care

Realizing that many people don't care about your organization may feel rotten. Coming to terms with this idea requires you to give up many of the illusions you may have had about connecting your organization to the general population. But don't worry, reconciliation and acceptance are possible and typically follow the path known as the five stages of grief. It might look something like this:

Stage One: Denial – "What do you mean Joe Public doesn't care about our hospital? How dare you! Who the *&^$ do you think you are? We save lives, we offer community benefit, we care about our patients, and we're awesome! Of course they care! Now good day sir. I said, good day!"

Stage Two: Anger – "Seriously, they don't care? Well then, screw them. Let them go somewhere else when they're bleeding out the ear. Really, after all we've done for this community, and now they don't care? Good luck with that type 2 diabetes diagnosis. You're on your own!"

Stage Three: Depression – "Wow, maybe they don't care? Really, they may not care about us? That's so awful – we've always been there for them. Maybe we haven't done enough? Maybe my billboards didn't really explain how awesome we are? If they don't care, what's the point of marketing to them? Why even bother? Maybe I'll just curl up here on the office couch and get some sleep. I don't think I can really go on."

Stage Four: Bargaining – "I'd do anything if they did care. I'll stop using pictures of all those docs in our print advertisements. I won't promote our colonoscopy services. I promise never to utter the phrases 'continuum of care' or 'high tech, high touch,' ever again. If only they would care about us."

Stage Five: Acceptance – "OK, so the majority of consumers in our market don't care about us. That's not the end of the world. That's the case for any number of businesses, including all of my competitors. I can still fulfill my role as a marketing leader and I can still help my organization achieve success. Let's face this challenge head on, and we'll be light years ahead of everyone else in achieving superior marketing performance. So where do I start?"

I've given the presentation titled "Joe Public Doesn't Care About Your Hospital" at numerous conferences, and because I'm primarily talking to healthcare marketers, most attendees are already at stage five, acceptance (though there are a few who linger in stage one, denial). But if the problem were convincing marketers of this truth, the sun would always shine, roses would always be in bloom, and all would be right with the world. Unfortunately, the challenge here is getting the rest of the organization on board with this reality. And that, my friends, can be a difficult task. Overcoming the challenge is crucial however, because embracing the concept that the majority of consumers in any given market don't care to hear from you will have profound implications on your marketing strategies.

What can you do if Joe Public doesn't care about your hospital?

At this point, you might be saying, "Gee whiz Chris, I think I buy into the idea that Joe Public doesn't care about my organization, but now what am I supposed to do?" Well, I'm glad you asked. For starters, as I've already alluded, the first strategy is to build your brand through a unique and compelling *experience*. Take Starbucks, one of the most powerful brands in the world. They created that brand leadership not through advertising, social media, or marketing communications, but by delivering a unique and compelling coffee experience (what CEO Howard Schultz called the "third place," a warm, inviting locale for people to hang out and enjoy their coffee, fashioned after European street cafes). Schultz and his team built that brand with *no* advertising, in fact, only using mass advertising in recent years. Same goes with the iPod from Apple, Facebook, and other leading brands. Think about healthcare – what is arguably the world's most respected healthcare brand? The Mayo Clinic. Mayo built its brand by delivering an unmatched clinical experience. Again with *no* advertising (they too have only just recently started to advertise).

The idea here is that by building a powerful brand with experiences, you will generate value in the form of positive word of mouth communications and recommendations, often cited as the number one factor for consumers when making a healthcare choice. Not only will Joe Public hear about you from friends, family members, co-workers and others he trusts, making it more likely he will retain that information, but building a strong brand in this way is the best way to ensure you'll be ready for Joe Public when he does need care.

Of course, while healthcare marketers may be the best equipped in the organization to *understand* branding, they typically cannot build brand on their own. Here's how I describe the scope of branding in "A Marketer's Guide To Brand Strategy:"

Branding is first and foremost about living a brand. Consider some of the ways a hospital potentially builds its brand with a patient who comes in for a routine check-up. The patient (and his or her family) will notice some or all of the following:

- *The convenience of parking at the hospital and whether there is a cost*

- *The cleanliness of the bathrooms*

- *The level of eye contact from the staff member at the information desk*

- *The simplicity of the way-finding*

- *The length of the wait before an appointment*

- *The friendliness of the nurse during a blood pressure check*

- *The amount of time a doctor spends in the exam room*

- *The clarity of the bill that arrives 15 days later[17]*

The point is, true brand building requires the efforts of the entire organization, though marketers can obviously play a key role. (More about that in Chapter 4.)

Be ready when Joe is ready

Looking beyond the monumentally difficult work involved in building a strong organizational brand, there are a lot of ways you, as a marketer, can help Joe Public when he needs care. Because that's the whole problem, right? If Joe doesn't need care, you can't just tell him about how great you are. But when he does need care, you better be ready, with the red carpet rolled out. That means having in place:

- Smart Search Engine Optimization and Search Engine Marketing strategies, so Joe can find you when he starts looking.

- A clear and effective website, so Joe can find the information he needs on your services.

- Effective call center capabilities so when Joe calls, someone connects him with the right resource, *right* away.

- A smart social media strategy, so you can respond to Joe, if he reaches out through Twitter or Facebook.

- A customer relationship management (CRM) system, so you can identify and connect Joe with information that will help him find the right care at the right time.

- An up-to-date mobile strategy that includes smartphone applications and mobile-optimized websites, so Joe has a smooth experience when he finds you on his smart phone or tablet (which, according to most experts, will happen more often than finding you from his computer, starting in 2014).

While many organizations spend so much time, money and effort trying to woo Joe Public with the wrong messages and in the wrong ways, consider how much work could be done to better respond to Joe when he's ready to come to you.

Building both a differentiated and compelling experience, and ensuring you're ready for Joe when he's ready for you, are *reactive* strategies. That means you're primarily inwardly focused, preparing yourself for when Joe shows up on your doorstep, so you can react the right way. But what if you want to be proactive, and go knock on Joe's door? Can you do that if he doesn't care?

Building relevant messages with inbound marketing

The key to connecting with Joe Public can be summarized in one word: ***relevance***. *To connect with Joe Public, you must make your message relevant.* That means moving beyond "me-first" messaging featuring your doctors, your technology and your awesomeness. There are any number of ways you can deliver relevant messages, whether it's through compelling patient stories or creative angles that draw in audiences. Perhaps one of the best ways to accomplish this feat is through inbound marketing.

In 2009, I had the weird experience of stumbling upon a piece of jargon I hadn't heard before, but which described a concept I knew quite well. The term was "inbound marketing." (The concept is close to Seth Godin's "permission marketing," but I stopped reading after his 37th book, so maybe that's why I missed it.) According to the Hubspot Inbound Internet Marketing blog, inbound marketing is defined as "marketing focused on getting found by customers." This is the opposite of traditional, or "outbound marketing," with its goal of finding customers.[18] (Or what Godin calls "interruption marketing.") In this model, instead of pushing your message out to potential customers to compel them to try your product or service, you create content of one kind or another that pulls people in and makes them want to find out about you. Instead of running TV commercials, it's posting videos people want to share on YouTube. Instead of a print ad, it's a blog. In a way, it's the difference between quantity and quality. With outbound marketing, the quantity of impact is usually measured, and more is always better. (Think of the millions of impressions you might get from a mass advertising campaign.) With inbound marketing, your goal is far fewer contacts, but those contacts are of much higher quality because they want to connect with you. So while the numbers may be lower, the effort is more effective, because you've spent far less money for more qualified contacts.

For years, we've been advocating that hospitals and health systems pursue inbound marketing, we just didn't call it that. When we stress you need to remember consumers are driven by "what's in it for me," we're invoking the concept. When we suggest hospitals connect with consumers about "health" (something everyone is interested in) instead of "healing" (something only the sick are interested in), we're invoking the concept.

Building your brand with wellness

Consider the benefits of wellness-based messaging as an inbound marketing strategy. Most people don't need laser surgery or a new physician, so those ubiquitous messages don't resonate as well. It's not that you can't build brand with these messages – you can. But because they're not relevant to the vast majority of people in your community, it takes much more time and money for them to have an impact.

Most people do have some level of interest in living healthier lives, however, whether it's losing weight, cutting stress, exercising more, eating right, or whatever. A message focused on health and wellness is a message relevant to a lot more people, one that actually will build their awareness, along with their perception, utilization – and loyalty. And it's a message that's completely natural coming from a community health leader – *you*.

Wellness also helps deflect the negative focus on healthcare advertising. It's one thing to spend millions of dollars on advertising bragging about your awards or touting your new technology. It's quite another to be focused on helping those in the community improve their health and pursue wellness. This isn't a reason to focus on wellness as a brand message, but it's a nice side effect.

Finally, wellness messaging will actually help improve the health of your community. Anything we do as organizations from a marketing communications perspective that brings the right patient to the right service helps improve the health of consumers (assuming, of course, the right service is *your* service). As opposed to marketing messages focused on promoting the benefits of your organization, however, wellness-based messaging focuses on what's best for the audience, and is bound to help those in the community improve their health. So, not only is it the right thing to do from a business perspective, it's just the right thing to do, period.

There will be, of course, those in your organization who will argue you don't get "paid" for health and wellness, so why focus on it? There are some exceptions – helping diabetics meet certain benchmarks, for example, can be tied to better reimbursement from payers. But from a short-term perspective, that's mostly accurate – hospitals and physicians don't get paid for keeping people healthy (though healthcare reform regulations are supposed to eventually change that equation). Here's the disconnect: you will get paid

45

from promoting health and wellness, just not always today. When this argument comes up, use our old branding friend Starbucks to make your point. Imagine if the CEO of Starbucks had once said: "why should we invest in hiring friendlier baristas, or buying more comfortable furniture? We don't get paid for that, we get paid when people buy our coffee."

Seems kind of silly, right? People buy more coffee *because* of the investment in the Starbucks experience, and more people will engage your organization more times when you invest in the patient experience, or help them stay healthier with services, communications, education and more geared toward wellness. (Remember, the beauty of promoting health and wellness is that it's relevant to your audience, making them more likely to notice, listen, and engage when they need you.) It's not about getting paid today (though with the right wellness-based marketing, you will connect with those who *do* need care today), it's about getting paid *tomorrow*.

The good news is that we're seeing more hospitals and health systems attempt to build their brand on a position of health and wellness. The bad news is that if you're not one of those organizations, you may be left behind. You see, that's the Achilles heel of wellness as a brand position – anyone can claim it. Of course, like everything else (clinical quality, convenience, patient experience, advanced technology, etc.), how organizations actually deliver on this promise varies greatly. But unlike some of the other potential positions a provider could take, nearly every organization can pursue this position. And at some point, it could become ubiquitous in a given market, much as "we care," or "high-tech, high-touch," or "we're award-winning" have become.

The key is to jump out there first and stick with it. Not for six months, not for two years, but for a long, long time. Be the first, be the most, and be the best – don't just talk wellness, but build offerings and content that support the brand and that will consistently keep you ahead of the pack. Once you're out there, if you don't let up, it will be very difficult for others to catch you. Of course, if you let someone else get first dibs, the same can be said for you.

A wellness success story

In August 2010, Interval client Inova Health System (Falls Church, VA) launched "FitFor50," a wellness campaign aimed at engaging consumers in a preventive health program. The campaign featured former Washington Redskins football great Darrell Green as a passionate spokesperson, and provided a 50-day wellness program through FitFor50.org. The online experience included videos and tips from Darrell and Inova physicians, wellness content, and an interactive Wellness Playbook, which allowed registered users to log their own wellness goals and update their personal progress. (We designed the FitFor50.org website and interactive Wellness Playbook tool.) One month after launching, the FitFor50 website had more than 26,000 unique visitors, and more than 6,500 people had registered for the Wellness Playbook. This led to more than 1,700 new records in the organization's CRM system, and 3,541 updated records.

Inova's director of digital marketing & communications Chris Boyer has this to say: "The FitFor50 site also integrates a number of social media elements, including blogs, Facebook, Twitter and YouTube. We've made an effort to ensure users of the site can interact with the content whatever way is most comfortable for them."

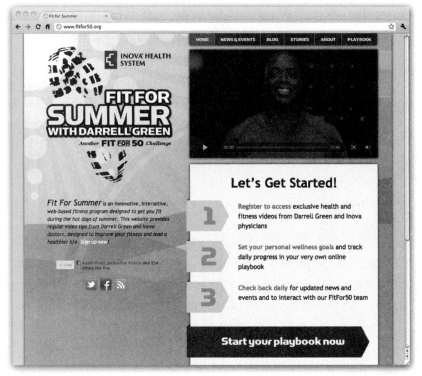

The FitForSummer campaign at FitFor50.org

The program continued in 2011 with updated online programs titled "FitForWinter," "FitForSpring," "FitForSummer" and more programs are planned for the future.

Boyer also offers this insight: "This program allowed for a much deeper interaction with participants. Why? Because wellness is relevant. Relevance turns interruption into appropriateness."

View the FitFor50 case study on ThinkInterval.com.

48

Just remember...

No matter how you approach this change – relevant messaging, wellness programs, or whatever – the key is to move your organization past the simplified and erroneous assumption that simply telling your market why you're great will lead to marketing results. If it helps, just keep repeating, "Joe Public Doesn't Care, Joe Public Doesn't Care, Joe Public Doesn't Care." Soon enough, that perspective will start to rub off on the right people.

CHAPTER TWO:

Out with the old, in with the new

From the WeeklyProbe:

Famous septuagenarian couple on tandem bike retires from stock photo career

The couple who made hospital and health system advertising familiar to so many across America is calling it a day. Steve Madson, 74, and his wife Sherry, 73, are the famous couple seen riding a tandem bike in so many hospital advertisements. They have graced billboards and newspaper ads in the healthcare world for more than three decades, but have recently decided to hang up the bike and retire.

"Good thing we weren't actually riding all those times the picture was used," joked Steve, a former barber. "We would have put a million miles on that bike!"

Steve and Sherry's introduction into healthcare advertising began in 1973, when Steve's brother, Brian, snapped a shot of the couple riding a tandem bike through Hyde Park in New York. Brian happened to work at a nearby hospital and brought the picture into work the following day, showing it around the department.

"Our corporate council really loved it, and we thought, why not use this to promote our hospital?" said Brian. "Who knew it would grow to become such a classic icon?"

Over the 35+ years since, Steve and Sherry have been photographed on more than 127 different tandem bikes and used in more than 1,400 hospital and health system ad campaigns. According to Steve, what started as something fun the couple did on the side turned into a lucrative business in the 1990s.

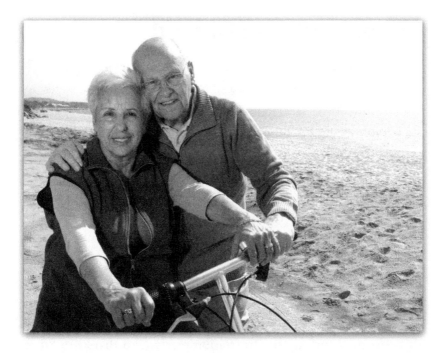

"That's when it really took off, thanks to the availability of cheap stock photography over the Internet," he said. "At that point, every hospital, system, clinic, doctor or veterinarian could use our photo. And it seemed like they did!"

Now independently wealthy, Steve and Sherry plan on traveling the world before settling down in their hometown of Miami, Florida.

"We probably could have kept going for years," Sherry said. "But it felt like it was time to move on to something new."

The bane of the billboard

If one word summarizes the problems with healthcare marketing today, it might very well be "billboard." As I reflected in the introduction of this book, the "billboards will solve everything" suggestion would be funnier if it didn't happen so universally, and so often.

Not that I have anything against billboards – we've created dozens. They obviously have a place in the universe of potential marketing tactics. But the clarion call of "let's put up a billboard" is one of the more obvious signs that hospital and health system marketing needs to shed its rudimentary, tired approaches and join other industries in embracing sophisticated and innovative marketing strategies. Recently, Steve Davis, a healthcare strategist, consultant, and author of the "Health Care Strategist" blog, wrote this post that sums up the frustration nicely (and thanks to Steve for letting me share it here):

"The mind reels and the eyes spin after a 1,000 mile cross-country drive. Why? Not for the traffic jams caused by Illinois' mind-numbingly stupid decision to waste "stimulus" dollars repaving an already perfectly-smooth I-55 from St. Louis to Joliet. You expect idiocy from Illinois politicians. And the paving contractor is probably some pol's brother-in-law.

No, my allergic reaction stems more from the astounding numbers of bad, really, truly, horribly, miserably, wretched billboards devoted to hospital marketing messages. C'mon people. What are you THINKING?

Dumb clients? Clueless agencies? One has to wonder.

Copy that rambles on...and on...and on. Can't ANYBODY get to the POINT in 6 words or less? Colors that wash out in the sun...and under sodium vapor lights...and at dawn...and dusk. Isn't someone paying for these things DRIVING THE BOARD once in a while?

Acronyms and buzzwords. Do you REALLY think a billboard is the place to be telling the masses about your smashing new EMR or your performance improvement activities? Really? Sorry, at 75 mph, when I see "PI" I think Magnum, not readmission rates.

Confusing names. "The Blah-Blah Institute at South MegaPlex Hospital & Medical Center's North Main Street Pavilion." All I get is "..Blah-Blah..." All I care about is...well, I don't care. I passed caring 10 miles ago. What's that you say? Cross-country drivers aren't really your intended audience? You're going after the locals? Yeah, maybe, but you're paying for BOTH. And you're reaching neither.

Next time I'm flying. Whatever's in American Airlines' seat-back pockets has to be easier on my eyes than what adjoins our interstate highways, though undoubtedly less rant-worthy. On second thought, who am I kidding?" [19]

Time to shake things up

Unfortunately, billboards are just one symptom of the disease that is old-school healthcare marketing. What else is old-school? "Look at us, aren't we great!" advertising. Poorly designed websites. Over-reliance on mass advertising. Sending press releases out en-masse. Launching massive campaigns with no thought of measuring success. The list goes on and on. What's new school? Mobile strategies to connect with patients, consumers and physicians wherever they are. Social media adoption. Inbound marketing and relevant content. Quick Response (QR) codes in ads. Location-based services. Talking with your audience instead of at them. Adopting sophisticated marketing strategies and tools, such as CRM, call centers and online patient portals. Search engine marketing. Building a marketing measurement discipline. This list also goes on and on.

Don't believe me when I say we're an industry stuck in the past? Consider these points of evidence:

- According to the IAB Internet Advertising Report conducted by PricewaterhouseCoopers and the Interactive Advertising Bureau, advertising expenditures on Internet advertising exceeded those of newspaper advertising for the first time in 2010.[20] Yet according to the latest "By The Numbers" report from SHSMD, healthcare marketers spent 24% of their advertising budget on print advertising, and only 5% on the Internet.[21] And according to J.K. Lloyd, president and co-founder of search engine marketing firm Eruptr and former executive at Revolution Health, 80% of hospitals have never used search engine marketing.[22]

- According to a list compiled by healthcare social media expert Ed Bennett, 1,188 U.S. hospitals have a Facebook page, 788 have a Twitter account, 548 have YouTube channels, and 137 have an organizational blog (as of June 2011).[23] (While Ed says the list likely misses some hospitals, it is recognized by many in the industry as one of the leading compilations of hospital social media activity). There are 6,000+ hospitals in the U.S., though some healthcare marketers believe many of those hospitals, for one reason or another, couldn't or shouldn't be using social media in a significant way. Yet even cutting that total in half, only one third of the remaining 3,000+ hospitals appear on Facebook (which has nearly 700 million global users and counting).

- According to Mary Meeker, former Morgan Stanley analyst who has been dubbed the "Queen of the Internet" by Barron's magazine for her prescient predictions of the Internet boom of the late 1990s, access to the Internet from smart phones and other mobile devices will exceed access from desktop browsers by 2014.[24] (Other experts have predicted this tipping point will come in 2013 or earlier with the advent of tablets like the iPad). Yet according to Paul Griffiths, CEO of healthcare web strategy firm MedTouch (and whom I shall dub the Duke of the Internet), their survey of the industry revealed that 20% of hospitals claim to have a mobile-optimized website and/or a mobile web application.[25] (An informal search of hospital websites seems to reveal that a much lower number *actually have* a mobile-optimized version of their organization's website.)

- Karen Corrigan, owner of Corrigan Partners, a 30-year veteran of healthcare marketing and one of the most respected voices in the industry, estimates that less than 25% of hospitals and health systems have marketing truly integrated as a core business competency.

- Based on my research for "The Marketer's Guide to Brand Strategy," I've estimated that less than 10% of hospitals or health systems are guided by an active *brand* strategy (as opposed to a naming strategy, or brand identity guidelines).[26] While branding has moved closer to the forefront since that time, it's likely a stretch to say that group now represents more than one fifth of all hospitals.

To truly break the chains of the past and rally to meet the challenges of the future, healthcare marketers must assess their old standby practices and outdated methods and embrace new ways of thinking and reaching their audiences. It starts with opening your mind and moving beyond the Hidden Gem Syndrome, accepting that Joe Public Doesn't Care About Your Hospital, and engaging consumers in a more relevant way. But there's so much more we can do. It's time to stop the madness, shake things up, and raise the bar of healthcare marketing by moving on from the tired old ways of the past.

Over-reliance on "old marketing"

In early 2011, I attended a national conference for healthcare marketers and communicators (the name of which I shall not disclose). During a conference lunch, a poll was projected on a large screen at the front of the room, which showed real-time responses as attendees texted their answers to the poll. (Now that's pretty new-school!) The problem was the poll itself, which asked "Where do you receive your healthcare news?" The following possible responses were given:

- television

- newspaper

- radio

- websites

- trade publications

- other

Hmmm, what's missing? Perhaps social media, which given the audience, would likely have been the number one answer. Not to pick on this organization, but the exclusion of social media in many ways represents the challenge our industry has with letting go of the past and moving forward.

58

The use of traditional media channels for promotion – such as television, print, and, yes, outdoor – still dominates the typical healthcare marketing plan, despite the erosion of viewers, readers and effectiveness of these channels. Many experts say "old marketing" – as defined by traditional paid advertising – is dead or dying in large part because consumers say they no longer want to be sold to or interrupted, that they want to have authentic engagements with brands, and to have a voice when it comes to engaging the companies from which they buy. Therefore, because consumers say they don't like the "old" methods that rely on interruption or selling, and because they have the means to avoid those methods, "old marketing" is no longer effective. In support of this viewpoint, research has shown the migration away from these means by consumers, such as in the drop in network television viewing – and the resulting drop in ad views – thanks to the proliferation of segmented television content, online content, technology like TiVo, and more.

I've spent a lot of energy in our blog, podcasts and speaking engagements trying to make the case for why healthcare marketers should move away from the reliance on "old marketing" and pursue strategies such as building authentic brand experiences, embracing transparency, leveraging social media, expanding interactive engagement and more. To be fair, I don't really think "old marketing" is dead just yet. I don't think people ever wanted to be sold to or interrupted (for the most part). It's just that during the rise of advertising and mass media starting in the 1950s, there was no other way for marketers to reach them, so that's what they did. Even though consumers really weren't thrilled with it, they couldn't avoid it, so mass advertising was effective essentially by default. Today, consumers say they don't want to be sold to, and they say they don't want to be interrupted, and research shows how they're avoiding this wherever they can. But whether they believe it or not, whether they would admit it or not, whether they would even know it or not, mass media still does impact consumers when it reaches them. It may not be the preferred or most effective method in many cases, but the stuff still has an effect.

The problem isn't that "old marketing" isn't effective (though by almost any measure it's definitely dropping in effectiveness). The problem is that these methods are overused by healthcare marketers when more effective strategies are available. Why spend hundreds of thousands of dollars on a service line advertising campaign without first maximizing your referring physician efforts? Why erect a dozen billboards when your website is clunky? The trick is finding the right balance between "old" and "new" marketing, using each to support the other, and mixing the spend and effort in a way that maximizes impact.

Broaden your creative thinking

For starters, healthcare marketers can expand how they think about creativity when it comes to marketing.

Last summer, I was able to catch up with the rest of the world by watching the first three seasons of the hit TV show *Mad Men* on DVD. The show is a marvel on many levels, but given my position in the world of marketing, I was particularly drawn to the scenes when Don Draper, creative director at the Sterling Cooper ad agency and the show's protagonist, presented creative ideas to clients. Certainly Don was a force of charisma and confidence, practically bending clients to his will. What was startling, however, was the continuous simplicity of the big ideas Don presented. Maybe it was a clever headline, or compelling artwork, or a memorable theme, but creative was always presented in the context of a print ad, or, at a higher level, a television spot. No matter the client or the product, the big idea was always a form of advertising.

Now contrast that with today's world. Certainly captivating advertising is still part of the mix. But now, creativity can be applied to a healthcare marketing challenge on so many levels. Visionary concepts can come in the form of an innovative media strategy, or the enterprising use of specific channels, such as social media or mobile technology. Online strategies are rife with creative opportunity, from interactive websites to iPhone apps. Healthcare marketers can drive breakthrough ideas in service innovation or enhanced patient experiences, or by understanding and approaching new markets in new ways. At the highest level, marketers can pull multiple components together in imaginative strategies, combining a new experience with a twist on an important customer segment, mixed with clever social media components. As an example, consider the popular Old Spice Guy campaign. The advertising, featuring a macho spokesman as "The Man Your Man Could Smell Like," with hilarious, over-the-top spots, was considered extraordinarily creative, with videos that went viral and were seen millions of times on YouTube.[27] But the company took creativity to a new level when it hosted an "Ask the Old Spice Guy" event on Twitter, where followers could post questions and the Old Spice Guy would answer his favorites through quickly shot videos that were posted nearly real-time on Twitter.

Some may harken back to Don Draper's environment and dream wistfully of the simplicity of creativity in that earlier time. It's true that today's world, with all of its options for creativity, may seem complex or confusing to many healthcare marketers. But those who pursue creativity in all its potential forms, on all its many levels, will see that the opportunities to break through with new ideas have increased exponentially. Put another way, imagine what Don Draper could have done with Facebook!

Risks worth taking

Part of the problem with embracing the new world of marketing and communications is the generally conservative nature of our industry. The healthcare industry is, by its very nature, risk averse: Think Hippocratic Oath, the essence of which is "First, do no harm." This is understandable from a clinical perspective, of course. But from a business perspective, taking strategic risks is how many organizations separate themselves from the pack. And now more than ever, hospitals and health systems need to consider taking strategic risks in how they market their services and build their brands.

To ensure their organization not just survives but thrives in today's challenging environment, healthcare marketers must embrace and execute brave new marketing strategies. This means finding new ways to establish genuine connections with today's savvy healthcare consumers and spur them to action. Executives who want to set their organizations apart must become willing to allow marketers to take calculated marketing and branding risks. Even with corner-office support, embracing the necessary risk will likely require a change in everyone's thinking and willingness to let go of old school approaches that simply don't register as well with consumers anymore.

Defining and embracing risk

Given the current market dynamics, what types of risks are worth taking, and how do you manage them? When it comes to healthcare marketing strategies and tactics, risks come in three different flavors – comfort, effectiveness and political.

Comfort risks

Because many administrative and clinical leaders in healthcare do not have extensive education or experience when it comes to marketing, they are most comfortable doing what they see others in the industry doing, whether it's effective or not. Unfortunately, this leads to "in-breeding" when it comes to marketing strategy in healthcare: everyone is doing the same thing, often with tactics that have little relevancy or impact. (I cover more on "Me Too" marketing in Chapter 3.)

Going out on a limb with something new or different is often the hardest risk for leaders to embrace. But breaking free from the comfort-zone is often what it takes to stand out in a crowded market, change perceptions, or capture new audiences. Consider HealthPartners, the Minnesota-based health system that launched a campaign to promote preventive care and diagnostic testing using mascot-like characters that included a six-foot tall urine sample cup called "Petey Pee Cup." Imagine the angst during the approval process for hitting the market with something so bold, so *different*.

Other examples of breaking out of the traditional comfort zone include advertising campaigns that run an upfront teaser phase – with no organizational logo or name – to generate buzz, or the use of humor in healthcare advertising. Or being one of the first to create an "Emergency Room Wait Time" iPhone app, as Inova Health System did in 2010.

Managing comfort risks takes patience. Persuading people to move beyond their comfort zones in a significant way doesn't happen overnight. If you're taking this kind of risk, build in plenty of time for review and discussion, and expect a "two steps forward, one step back" style of progress. Leverage whatever evidence, outside expertise or case studies you can to help bolster your case.

Effectiveness risks

Marketers in all industries, healthcare included, are being asked to demonstrate the ROI of their strategies. "Why should we spend $300,000 on this campaign? How many patients will we draw? What is the downstream revenue we can expect? How do we measure results?" This trend is actually great for marketers, as it will allow them to demonstrate their true value to their organizations. (We'll talk more about this in Chapter 5.) But the call for ROI is sometimes a disguise for risk aversion. For those unwilling to take the risk, it's easy to hide behind the phrase "If you can't prove the ROI, then it's not worth doing." The problem with this thinking is summed up in a quote from Albert Einstein, who we would think, as a scientist, would be the last to question the value of empirical evidence. He said:

"Not everything that can be counted counts, and not everything that counts can be counted."

This quote helps explain why an organization might pursue activities where the exact effectiveness may be unknown, or not easily measured. It also reflects the spirit of innovation the process of bringing something brand new to the market – something that by definition will have no track record of success (or failure), because there's never been anything like it. Consider the first mini-clinics. Certainly, the folks behind MinuteClinic – the first mini-clinic business in the U.S. – had a business plan that predicted certain revenue, patients, profit and more. But they couldn't be certain of their success, as there was nothing that existed with which to compare it. Someone had to be willing to take a chance on the idea and risk failure by investing capital and energy investment to launch that new business model.

Another great example of pursuing a marketing strategy where effectiveness is unknown is the use of social media as part of a marketing plan. Creating a page on Facebook or having clinical leaders communicate through Twitter are tactics that those in our industry are still trying to understand from a value perspective. But these new channels may provide exciting opportunities for providers, and those who find ways to successfully leverage these types of social networks first will benefit the most.

In general, it's a good policy to be upfront and honest about whatever risk is at hand, but it is especially important when managing effectiveness risks. For example: "This is new, so we're not 100% certain of success. But given our projections and built-in contingencies, we estimate a $500,000 investment that has a 20% likelihood of breaking even, and a 60% change of delivering positive ROI."

Political risks

By political, we mean internal politics, or the power many in the organization hold over marketing strategies (whether or not they should hold that power). It's amazing how often marketing strategies are pursued primarily because someone in the organization – typically a physician, but sometimes an administrative leader – demands it, not because it's the smart or effective thing to do. We've actually had CEOs say to us and their marketing leaders, "I know it's not going to work, but do it anyway." Why? Because there is often a political risk in upsetting a key surgeon who's demanding a series of billboards to promote his general surgery practice. The risk is in creating an adversarial relationship with these powerful physicians, and given the deeper issues confronting leadership when it comes to physician relations (authority, processes, pay), giving in on marketing decisions is often seen as a path of least resistance.

It can be very difficult for hospital and health system leaders – let alone marketing leaders – to take a risk and stand up to this pressure. But doing so will often lead to more effective solutions and better results. We've found that taking political risks in healthcare marketing is often the most difficult form of risk taking, and suggest doing so in small doses. For example, set a goal that in year one, you'll give in to 80% of the "political" requests, but stand up to 20%. Often, a straightforward and honest discussion with physicians, clarifying the true goals of marketing efforts (new patients, increased volumes, etc.), along with an explanation of why certain approaches work, goes a long way.

Take the lead

In the current economic and regulatory climate, no organization can afford to keep doing things the way they've always been done. The time has come where willingness to try new things is almost no longer optional – it's rapidly becoming critical. If healthcare providers are to thrive, it will be in large part as a result of tenacious marketers, those who understand the true value of marketing and branding pushing the boundaries and taking risks to benefit the industry, your organization and consumers alike.

Take it from Richard S. Tedlow, a professor of business administration at Harvard Business School, who said in a 2009 Businessweek article: "A leader is someone who doesn't do what everyone else does."[28]

A different perspective on physicians in advertising

One of the ways I'm constantly imploring healthcare organizations to shake things up is to move beyond the clichéd advertising that seems so prominent in our industry. Ads featuring awards, anything with the words "we care," a picture of a 60-something couple on a tandem bike, or physicians and nurses in their white coats are among the most painful.

That said, even the worst cliché positioned in the right context can work. Susan Solomon, vice president of marketing at St. Joseph's Health System in Orange, California, weighs in here.

"I believe so much hospital advertising is too impersonal, focused on 'centers of excellence' or big white shining buildings," Solomon says. "But using physicians in your advertising in the right way can have tremendous benefits."

Doctors have the most credibility with consumers, says Solomon, and make excellent spokespeople for hospitals and health systems.

"One aspect of health reform moving forward is the idea that people should spend less and less time in hospitals, so it makes sense to start leveraging those relationships that will always be central to healthcare – the physician-patient relationship," Solomon says.

Solomon also notes that physicians can provide a local tie-in that helps distinguish a hospital or health system. So much hospital advertising is so generic, she says, it could be plopped down in any market and still make sense. Bringing physicians forward as individuals can really help differentiate an organization. As an example, Solomon cites a campaign she developed for MemorialCare Medical Centers based in Long Beach, California, which leveraged physicians as spokespeople for the system in a comprehensive television advertising campaign. She says the campaign ran for nearly 10 years and had great results, including high recall among consumers and strong support among the medical staff.

"The physicians featured in the ads were really passionate in delivering the messages, and they really stayed on point," Solomon says. "Plus, working hand in hand with physicians to create the campaign had its own benefits, such as more support from the medical staff for marketing efforts and a better working relationship between marketing and physicians."

Solomon acknowledges that if not done well, using physicians in hospital advertising can make it tough to differentiate a hospital, especially in a market with a high-level of physician-based advertising. She says it helped that physicians typically aren't highlighted in the Los Angeles market, but no matter the market, the key is presenting physicians as individuals.

"People can connect with certain kinds of physicians, such as primary care doctors, who they have an ongoing relationship with. You just need to bring them forward as people – individuals – so they're accessible," notes Solomon. "Remember, we're marketing a human service after all."

CHAPTER THREE

Break
bad habits

From the WeeklyProbe:

Standing up to doc leads to marketer performing aortic valve repair surgery

A routine business meeting at Evergreen Hospital ended with the vice president of marketing agreeing to perform heart surgery. The move followed a heated discussion on the merits of a marketing tactic suggested by a heart surgeon.

Janet Nolan, MD, a cardiovascular surgeon, was advocating for printing advertising on java jackets (coffee cup wraps) to help address a persistent lag in cardiology consults.

"Everyone drinks coffee, and many will eventually require cardiovascular intervention," said Dr. Nolan. "And think of all the caffeine-induced arrhythmias we'd be in front of. The strategy is so obvious it makes you question the intelligence of our marketing staff."

Vice President of Marketing Ted Beech tried to counter Dr. Nolan by stressing the referral-driven nature of cardiac care, as well as the high cost of printing thousands of custom coffee cup wraps compared with the minimal conversion rate. Finding no flexibility from Dr. Nolan, Beech played the logic card:

"Look, I don't tell you how to perform heart surgery," said Beech. "Why won't you trust that I know what's best when it comes to marketing?"

Shocking those in attendance, Dr. Nolan offered to let Beech perform surgery if he would consider the coffee cup wrap strategy. Feeling he had to step up to the challenge, Beech agreed. He has been scheduled to perform a normally simple aortic valve repair on a 52-year old male early next week.

"Of course I'm terrified," said Beech, explaining that unfortunate provisions of HIPAA actually preclude him from warning the patient of this unprecedented move. Staff have coined the switch "Dare to Care" after administration rejected a "Freaky Surgery Friday" moniker. If the surgery is successful, Beech has promised to print 500,000 coffee cup wraps with the slogan "Considering heart surgery? Sip the best service around at Evergreen Hospital."

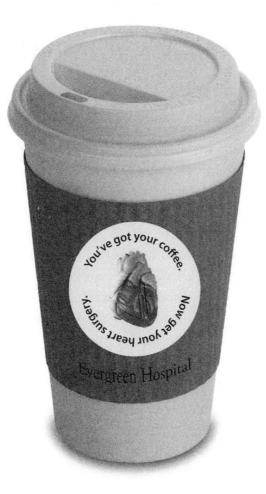

The first two chapters of this book explore two critical shifts in thinking – moving beyond the "just tell them" mentality, and letting go of the old and embracing the new. But adopting these two philosophies won't be enough to move our industry forward in a significant way. We also have to break some of our most persistent bad habits when it comes to marketing. The five habits I call out here are so common, it's likely every healthcare marketer has dealt with them at some level (I've already referenced a few in earlier pages). The fact that they're recognizable doesn't make them easier to break, of course. But we can do it – I know we can!

Habit One – "Little M" marketing

Much of healthcare marketing today is really focused on what might be called "Little M" marketing, which really means marketing communications. While there is obviously a role for this level of marketing, too much emphasis on communications holds marketers back from truly impacting their organizations.

In one of the classic definitions of marketing, there are four "P's" – product, price, place and promotion. Most healthcare marketers are only focused on one of those "P's" – promotion. Two of the great minds in healthcare marketing – David Marlowe and Karen Corrigan – are of one voice on this subject: Marketing is more than just marketing communications.

"Marketing is far more than the brochure of the week," says Marlowe, principal, Strategic Marketing Concepts (and someone I consider to be the "godfather" of healthcare marketing). "The marketing department should be doing much more than communications – access, experience, pricing, etc. And much of marketing for a hospital actually takes place from outside of the marketing department, in the delivery of the patient experience. And that's a good thing."

Part of the issue, says Marlowe, is that many professionals who are responsible for marketing at hospitals and health systems have a communications or public relations background, which can lead to an overemphasis on that component of the marketing mix.

"As the old saying goes, to a man with a hammer, everything looks like a nail," he says. "CEOs are frustrated because they know marketing is about more than running an ad, but they are not sure what it should be. And they don't see their marketers stepping forward and filling that void."

Here's how 30-year healthcare marketing vet Karen Corrigan from Corrigan Partners describes the dilemma:

"Marketing is a core business competence, just like supply chain management, finance, or any other key discipline," says Corrigan. "And that requires an executive team that focuses marketing strategy on creating real value for the organization. If marketing is not aligned with and supporting the core business strategies, it limits marketing to a tactical level, and you're missing the boat."

The bad news? As noted in Chapter 2, Corrigan estimates (generously, she says), that less than 25% of organizations truly have marketing integrated as a core business competency. She thinks that maybe another 25% at least get this concept, but haven't invested in the expertise or systems to make it happen.

Corrigan also notes: "There are a whole host of activities that fall under marketing's realm that aren't about driving growth at all. Who's responsible for creating the hand-washing posters? The marketing department. But what's that got to do with building a market?"

Of course, the key to moving away from "Little M" marketing to a more strategic, holistic "Big M" marketing discipline is organizational leadership.

Without the support of leaders who understand and value marketing at its true level it will be very difficult for healthcare marketers to demonstrate the true value of marketing discipline. The overemphasis on communications, for example, often comes from leaders who don't recognize the totality of marketing, according to Corrigan.

In fact, I think it's safe to say great healthcare marketing cannot happen without great leadership.

It starts at the top

In my observations over the past 12 years in healthcare marketing, there is one ingredient that is essential to sustained marketing success: great organizational leaders. CEO, president, administrator – the title doesn't matter. Time and time again I have seen sophisticated, cutting edge and effective marketing strategies fail to get off the ground due to lack of support from the organizational leader.

Providing healthcare services in today's market is an extraordinarily difficult proposition. Leaders must firmly grasp clinical operations, financing, regulations, physician relations, labor relations, clinical quality and safety dynamics, and much more. Marketing and branding is – and maybe should be – farther down on the list of skill sets for organizational leaders. However, in today's market, with rising consumerism, increased competition, transparency and more, successful marketing and brand building is vital to long-term sustainability and so leaders either need to acquire more marketing and branding acumen – or hire healthcare marketing talent they trust to fill the gap.

Given these limitations, how would I define a great leader in terms of supporting effective "Big M" marketing? Here are four main qualities:

1. A great leader understands the value of brands, and more importantly, understands strong brands are built primarily through the experience offered, not through advertising or communications. With that understanding, they support the investment in and often long-term incubation of service innovation and enhanced patient experiences. On the flip side, they don't ask marketing leaders to use advertising campaigns to "build our brand" or "fix our reputation." Says Corrigan: "Healthcare organizations are often so operationally focused, they see the world from the inside out. Leaders should embrace a customer-centric philosophy, as well as understand what drives competitive strategy and how they can affect change in the market."

2. A great leader is able to look beyond what their peers are doing and take risks, or try new approaches. The healthcare industry is notorious for looking across the street to see what others are doing, then following. When it comes to marketing, however, this leads to a vicious cycle of outdated or ineffective practices replicated over and over. A great leader is open to ideas new to healthcare – often from other more advanced industries – even when it seems peers aren't pursuing the strategy.

3. A great leader is able to stand up to physicians or others who play power politics and push for bad marketing. Leaders often are worn down by various physician relation issues – authority, process, compensation, etc. – so they give on

marketing or branding issues. The political power play is perhaps the number one reason effective marketing dies on the vine.

4. A great leader understands marketing and branding, but if not, then trusts her marketing leader. We shouldn't expect all healthcare leaders to have a total grasp of all the functions they oversee – that's why they have experienced leaders in each area. But if the leader doesn't trust her lieutenant when an "understanding gap" exists, what's the point? When the marketing leader is advocating in any of the situations noted above, the organizational leader must have his back as often as possible.

A simple way to move beyond "Little M" marketing

As I've shown, for marketers to demonstrate the ultimate value of their discipline, they must move beyond the promotional level and begin to participate in – if not drive – discussions of price, patient experience, service levels and more. One way marketers can take that step is by embracing service innovation. What's service innovation? Here's how I described the concept in a paper titled "Competitive Differentiation Through Innovation." Though written in 2006, the definition still holds true today:

"Tom Kelly, a partner at leading design firm IDEO, perhaps captured it best: Focus on the kind of innovation where you 'passionately pursue new ways to serve your customers.' In business, what Kelly was referring to has been termed 'service innovation' to distinguish it from 'product innovation.' Rather than innovation related to a tangible product (like four-wheel drive technology on a car), service innovation is related to the business of how the car is sold (like no-haggle pricing first introduced by Saturn). In healthcare, that means distinguishing

between innovations related to the clinical care (the product) and innovations related to the business of providing healthcare. For marketers, these innovations also must provide a distinct competitive advantage. "[29]

How can a healthcare marketer embrace service innovation? My answer – use the iPod Mindset. In other words, think experience, and think *small*.

Rule 1: Think experience

Remember when the iPod first hit the scene in 2001? It was one of the most successful product launches of all time. Why? The greatest reason for the iPod's phenomenal success was the unbelievable *experience* Apple created for its users.

From the product's beautiful design, to its ease of use, to the revolutionary iTunes website that allowed consumers to buy and download songs for only 99 cents, the iPod experience was both compelling and different. The technology that allowed users to download, save, and play digital music was around well before the iPod. If the technology alone were responsible for the iPod's success, other MP3 music players might have enjoyed the same results – but they didn't.

What about advertising? Perhaps you remember the ubiquitous advertising for the iPod, featuring silhouetted figures dancing joyfully to hip music. But the iPod was a cultural icon *before* this campaign hit full stride. What drove the iPod's amazing success initially was the word of mouth buzz generated by the experience of using the iPod.

The next time you are asked to develop a marketing plan for a service line, or a promotional strategy for a program, or an ad campaign for a new clinic, ask yourself this: How can I make what

I'm promoting feel like an iPod? That is, how can I take what I am marketing, promoting, or advertising and create an experience that is both compelling and different?

Rule 2: Think small

Healthcare organizations often focus on experience improvement initiatives such as lean manufacturing, customer service training, facility upgrades, or technological improvements like the electronic medical record. Although all of these are powerful, long-term ways to improve the patient experience, they represent massive investments in organizational change. The iPod teaches us a lesson that can help healthcare marketers drive innovation in experiences their organization provides in a different way. One of the celebrated features of the iPod, of course, was its size – originally it was touted with the phrase "10,000 songs in a deck of cards." So, in looking for ways to innovate, remember Rule 2 of the iPod mindset: think *small*. Innovating on a smaller scale – a screening, program, class or service versus organization wide, multi-year initiatives with big budgets – will allow you to bring about change faster, more easily, and with more immediate results. Additionally, the success of one new experience can lead to the development of the next new experience. By creating new and better experiences, you will enable your organization to make an immediate impact on this new competitive world in days or weeks, instead of having to wait for the results of systemwide changes that could take months or years.

For example, a number of years ago we worked with North Memorial Hospital, a 500+ bed trauma center in Minneapolis that was opening the region's first women's heart clinic. Initial success of the clinic would be measured by the number of women seen for a standard heart disease screening, based on the potential

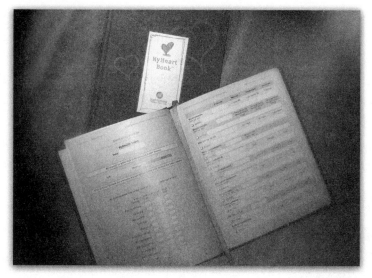

MyHeart Book

downstream care this would trigger. The marketing challenge, however, was how to distinguish the heart disease screening in a market saturated with similar offerings.

In our collaboration with the client, we hit on the idea of re-engineering the screening itself to create a differentiated and compelling offering.

The result was a one-of-a-kind, personalized experience called MyHeart Book. Women who participate in the program receive a personalized, hard-bound copy of MyHeart Book. The contents include the results of their assessment, 80+ pages of educational information, and a list of action steps developed in one-on-one interviews with a clinic staff member that includes diet and exercise recommendations, stress management techniques and more. The results from this innovative approach were immediate and significant. Within one month of opening, the clinic had booked more than 500 women five months in advance for the MyHeart Book program, a self-referred program with 100% of the $85 cost

81

borne by the consumer. The high demand for the service resulted in the clinic expanding to serve patients five days a week, from the original schedule of three days a week when it first opened. And perhaps the ultimate measure of success? The physicians begged the marketing team to suspend advertising MyHeart Book, given the high demand for the service. More than six years later, MyHeart Book continues to serve as a differentiated offering for the North Memorial Women's Heart Clinic.

View the MyHeart Book case study on ThinkInterval.com.

Stories like this can be found throughout the healthcare world – the Seaside Imaging Center in Celebration, Florida, the development of a culture of innovation at Memorial Health System in South Bend, Indiana, and Mayo Clinic's SPARC innovation lab – are all classic examples of service innovation in action. More recently, hospitals and health systems are delivering service innovation through online tools and experiences.

More on moving past 'Little M' marketing

There are any number of ways healthcare marketers can break the chains of "Little M" marketing, and driving service innovation is just one of them. For example, the drive toward Accountable Care Organizations (ACOs) and fee-for-performance offers a new perspective for marketers to consider, says Keith Jennings, a friend, fellow blogger and "ranter," and corporate communications executive at Jackson Healthcare, (Atlanta, GA).

Jennings asserts, "ACOs will benefit most when patients stay within the system, which means that volume growth, patient compliance and physician strategies will be essential." He says, "These are marketing opportunities at their core."

Taking this idea further: If your organization is part of an ACO, what will your branding strategy be? How will your organization fit (or not fit) within the ACO's brand? Will you have distinct marketing messages and efforts? How will each organization leverage the other, without causing confusion in the market?

These are questions that are made for "Big M" marketing thinking. Pricing strategy, service innovation, reform-based strategies – there are plenty of opportunities for healthcare marketers to contribute in a strategic way. But no matter which paths you choose, it should be clear: the more you and your team embrace "Big M" strategies, the more value you'll bring to your organization.

Habit Two – Politically driven marketing

I once worked with a hospital marketing director who was trying to manage the high-pressure demands of one of the organization's key physicians. No amount of advertising was ever enough, and the doctor's idea of what constituted "effective" marketing focused, shockingly, on himself as the star of the campaigns. When the marketing director finally pushed back with alternative strategies for accomplishing the physician's goal (which was, at least explicitly, more patient visits), the doctor went straight to the organization's CEO and complained.

Can you guess what happened next? If you're like many healthcare marketers, you know the sad tale all too well. The CEO went to the marketing director and said, "Give him what he wants. I don't care whether it's actually effective or not – just keep him off my back."

Take a look at your last marketing campaign or initiative. Most likely, the documented goals were something like: "improve awareness" or "increase volumes" or some other marketing-related metric. Now, how many of your goals looked like this:

- "Appease chief surgeon."

- "Apply CEO's favorite photography style."

- "Make employees feel better about themselves."

- "Get cardiologist/ortho service line director/whack board member out of our hair."

Yet, how many of you can honestly say that one of these "hidden" goals – or one close to it – didn't play a role in the marketing initiative? How many of you would admit that one of these hidden goals was actually the driving force behind your initiative?

It's the dirty little secret in healthcare marketing. So much of what hits the streets by way of marketing initiatives, especially advertising campaigns, is driven not by sound marketing strategy but in response to internal political pressure. In fact – many of the bad habits cited in this book – "old school" marketing, "Me Too" marketing, Whack-a-Mole marketing – are often driven primarily by politically driven marketing requests.

What's a politically driven marketing request? An initiative prompted not by goals intended first and foremost to drive marketing or business success, but by personal power, preferences or pressures. Some other examples include:

- A physician who wants to advertise because he saw a competing group advertise (or a physician with whom he went to medical school) on a billboard.

- An administrator who wants to tout each and every award that comes down the pike, regardless of whether it is distinguished or differentiating.

- A service line leader who wants to employ a tactic because their vendor – who is also a friend – is advocating for it.

- A nurse manager who wants to initiate a new marketing approach after a friend told her at the supermarket she was unaware of the manager's clinic.

- An executive who wants to buy advertising with a local media outlet because she serves on the same community charity board as the owner of the outlet.

- A CEO who rejects a corporate identity color option because it reminds him of a coat his wife used to have.

These are all actual examples of politically driven marketing requests I've encountered (yes, even the coat example – it was green, by the way). Undoubtedly, politically driven marketing decisions are found in any industry (as are politically driven decisions in other disciplines, such as finance or human resources). But that doesn't excuse the practice, or explain the high level of incidence within the healthcare marketing world. Imagine how much money, how many resources, and how much energy has been wasted to fulfill politically driven demands in healthcare marketing.

What can marketers do about this insidious affliction? It would be easy to advise you to "Just say no." But that's often not a realistic possibility. I've seen situations where marketing leaders try to stand up to such pressure, and are over time either ignored, marginalized, or in extreme cases, forced out. On the other end of the scale (or sometimes because of the real or implied threats tied to politically driven marketing requests), many marketers simply acquiesce, taking more of a CYA approach. But that typically results in more poor or misguided marketing or worse, encourages more of the unwanted behavior.

So what's the solution? Here are six ways to mitigate politically driven marketing requests:

1) Gain senior approval of marketing plans

Obviously, to gain approval of your marketing plan, you need to *have* a marketing plan. Unfortunately, many organizations don't. Your goal is to create a high-level plan that establishes the key marketing strategies for the year, provides general timelines for activities, and sets out budget allocations. The plan doesn't have to get into tactical detail – you can always create individual action plans for each initiative. The point is to put in writing your organization's marketing priorities, and have your leadership review and approve them.

While changes will need to be made to the plan as opportunities and challenges arise throughout the year, a policy should be adopted that requires senior-level approval of any change in high-level strategy or overall prioritization of efforts. With physicians, operational managers and others throughout the organization, this formalization of marketing priorities provides you a solid defense against politically driven requests. And when it's your leaders themselves who are making the requests (or supporting the requests of others), having this formalized plan and policy in place will make it a little more painful for them to override the organization's approved marketing priorities for political reasons.

2) Influence early

One of the problems with politically driven marketing requests is that once they're made, they're hard to circumvent. The executive or physician who makes the request may take your questions or push-back personally, or may see your case for an alternative strategy as a defensive play for power.

One way to diffuse these types of requests is to establish an ongoing marketing education program for internal leaders that includes administration, operational managers, and key physicians, and covers Marketing 101 topics such as understanding the intended audience, the pros and cons of various media channels, or how to fairly measure marketing initiatives. The primary goal of such a program: indoctrinate your organization with the right approach to marketing, thereby reducing the amount of ill-advised marketing ideas.

But the marketing education program serves another important purpose. By presenting your vision of the "right way" to market your organization, it provides you with a reference point for future discussions. So when Dr. Bighead demands a billboard featuring his smiling face, you can refer to the training session that covered "The power and limitations of outdoor advertising," which gives your argument more credibility and sounds less defensive. While such educational programs seem rare in the healthcare world, they are common in other industries.

3) Open a second front in your marketing war

When I spoke at a recent conference, an attendee offered her successful strategy for helping to deal with the politically-driven marketing request. She mentioned that when a certain doctor kept demanding an ad to promote an accolade he'd received, she worked with him to create a small print ad, letting him contribute ideas, copy changes and approvals along the way. The ad was small, so the expense was low. But she said the result was that the physician was happy, and she was able to limit the time, money, energy – and potentially negative impact – a larger effort would have entailed.

This is what I mean by opening a second front in your marketing war. The main battle line should be focused on the execution of legitimate strategies that will drive business success, build brand, increase volumes, create patient loyalty and more. But often, the politically driven marketing request runs counter to these goals. To minimize the distraction, consider opening up a second front, where you pull away as few of the resources as possible from the main front to placate the politically driven marketing requests. By meeting these requests, but minimizing their impact, you may still be able to retain enough resources to fight the main battle effectively. I realize that in some ways this sounds underhanded, or like you are playing a game with your leadership. In a perfect world, you wouldn't have to – they would trust your marketing expertise and you could drive marketing strategy the right way. But it's not a perfect world, and carefully placating some of these requests can be a safe middle ground between simply giving in, or fighting until the powers that be grow frustrated with you and find someone else who will give in.

4) Measure your marketing effectiveness

Perhaps the most effective way to fight politically driven marketing requests is to implement a sophisticated measurement discipline for your marketing strategies. (We'll talk about measurement in Chapter 5.) If you believe an executive or physician is barking up the wrong marketing tree, your best strategy is to prove your case. You can do that by measuring the impact of your marketing strategies over time, so you can learn – and show – what works and what doesn't. That way, the next time someone knocks on your door with a bad marketing concept you can defend your plan with data: "While I understand you'd like to run a full-scale advertising campaign to promote our new Obscure Vendor Quality Award, our measurement of such programs over the past few years has clearly demonstrated that promoting awards that aren't recognized by the community has little effect on our awareness and perception levels. Here is the data showing the results."

5) Let the sun shine in

Once you have a marketing plan, *share* it with the organization, preferably via your Intranet or a marketing department-specific microsite. (An alternative is to create a report or binder that's distributed to key constituents, such as executive leaders, operational directors or physicians.) In addition, as you activate your plan, be sure to update your site with completed activities and results. First, by sharing your marketing activities, you'll head off those who seem to think that if *they* don't know what's going on in marketing, then *nothing* must be happening in marketing. That state of mind is often the catalyst for a politically driven marketing request. Second, by reporting your results in a consistent and transparent way, you will begin to teach others in the organization what effective marketing looks like, hopefully heading off ill-advised ideas before they become a political force.

6) Help your CEO help you

To engage your CEO as an advocate in supporting your marketing decisions, it helps to walk a little in his or her shoes. Your CEO is trying to navigate the organization through dramatic industry changes such as healthcare reform, increased competition, demanding patients, increased regulations, decreased reimbursement, and more. Given this dynamic, marketing is typically not going to be her highest priority, making it more likely for her to give in on requests from others in the organization – whether they entail smart marketing decisions or not. Be respectful of the tough position your leader faces, and be reasonable in the battles you ask her to fight for you. Demonstrate how your recommendations are what's best for the organization, not just for you and your team.

No amount of planning or preparation will eliminate all politically driven marketing requests in your organization. But following these steps will definitely help you reduce their frequency and impact, allowing you to spend more of your time, energy and resources on the marketing initiatives that will actually have a positive effect on your organization.

Habit Three – "Me Too" marketing

Because so many healthcare executives don't understand marketing fully, they too often look to see what others are doing for a guide on how to market their own organizations. The same tired approaches are used over and over and over again, from straightforward patient testimonials – "Snowflake Hospital really cared for me" – to the use of supplier photography to promote new technology investments – "Popeye Clinics now offers the BS4000 triple-scan microfritter." I literally can't count the number of hospital ads I've seen promoting joint replacement surgery services with the headline "Get back in the swing of things" and a photo of a 70-something man or woman with a golf club.

Of course, just because your rival is pursuing a strategy doesn't make it right for you. And it doesn't make it necessarily effective, either. If it holds true that most healthcare organizations aren't following smart marketing strategies, then "Me-too" marketing simply leads to more bad marketing, or what I like to call "inbred" marketing.

To be fair, much of "Me Too" marketing stems from our industry's reliance on benchmarking and best practices. It makes perfect sense to track the best means for treating a disease or diagnosing a disorder – best practices improve the overall delivery of healthcare and saves lives. However, this attitude can bleed into our marketing efforts – if XYZ hospital is doing it, then we should be doing it, too. The difference, of course, is that the point of clinical benchmarking is that organizations become more alike. One of the primary goals of marketing, however, is to *differentiate* your organization from the competition. In the end, the more your marketing looks like your competitors, the worse off you're likely to be.

The battle of the gold stars

One of the most common ways in which healthcare organizations pursue "Me Too" marketing is in the promotion of awards and rankings. There are now dozens of sources rating hospitals for consumers, among them, Angie's List, Zagat's, HealthGrades, *U.S. News & World Report*, Thomson Reuters – the list goes on and on. But the problem with the awards and rankings that emanate from these sources is not with the accolades. It's akin to the NRA's stance on gun control: "Guns don't kill people, people kill people." With hospital awards, the awards don't make for bad marketing, *misused and over-abused awards promotion* makes for bad marketing.

To be fair, in some cases, an advertising campaign featuring a new award makes sense. Most times, however, it doesn't. It's not that awards can't help build a brand – they certainly can, and research in healthcare and other industries supports that notion. But from our perspective, while awards and rankings are a reasonable supporting benefit point, providers should think twice about making them the focus of marketing efforts. Here's why:

"Look at me, I'm Sandra Dee."

Awards are evidence (at least in most cases) of strong work in the organization, whether it's clinical, service-driven or other. When used as a supporting point in a marketing effort, awards lend legitimacy to claims of excellence. But when awards are the *focus* of the marketing effort, the promotion can become an exercise in self-aggrandizement. As I stressed in Chapter 1, marketing should always strive to start from the consumer and work backwards, remembering to answer the question, "What's in it for me?" Promoting awards usually means starting with the organization and working back to the consumer, which is a harder connection to make. As we've already noted, Joe Public – the majority of your consumer audience – doesn't need your hospital, so they don't care about your hospital ratings either. There's nothing in it for them.

"Here today, gone tomorrow."

Most awards and rankings apply to a limited timeframe, such as "Top Hospital of the Year," or "Best Service in 2010." But what sounds great today might invite questions tomorrow if your award doesn't continue. Sometimes you'll see organizations promoting something like this: "Best wait times in the metro area in 2002, 2004 and 2007." Without consistency, the impact of the ranking or award is lessened.

"The pick and choose principle."

Highlighting that you've won awards in '03 and '07, but not '04, '05, '06 or '08 is an example of the Pick and Choose principle. This is where only certain aspects of accolades are promoted, conveniently leaving out other aspects. Sometimes you see this with patient satisfaction surveys, where a hospital is ranked high in a certain area, such as housekeeping or food service. It's ok to promote accolades for specific areas, but be certain that the focus doesn't draw attention to what areas didn't receive recognition.

"The throw a rock in any direction, hit an awards-based hospital ad theory."

Anytime you're using a strategy that everyone else is using – "Me Too" marketing – the impact of that strategy diminishes. This is especially true in a crowded market, with multiple organizations promoting the same award, like the Thomson Reuters 100 Top Hospital Award. Sometimes, the award is for something different (like cardiac vs. oncology). Sometimes, it's a 2010 award vs. a 2011 award. These days, with so many awards, ratings and rankings, it seems every organization has at least one accolade to promote, and many have a slew. All of the shiny medals and crystal trophies start blending together quickly, rendering any attempt at differentiation fruitless.

"Consumers don't have a clue."

OK, that's a strong statement. Some consumers definitely have a clue. And some consumers have half-a-clue. But many consumers don't have a clue in understanding or differentiating between rankings and awards. This is why in many larger markets, the release of the HCAHPS patient satisfaction data barely made a ripple. How many of your neighbors have any idea what HCAHPS is? Or who Thomson Reuters is, for that matter?

This may change, of course, as consumer-driven healthcare spreads and more patients become responsible for how they spend their healthcare dollars. But at the same time, this trend is leading to the proliferation of these rankings and awards. There are probably more websites available now for ranking hospitals than there are for ranking cars. In an article in the *Colorado Springs Gazette* called "The Benefits of Making the Grade," the journalist starts off by saying, "When *Motor Trend* magazine releases its top picks for new cars and trucks each year, consumers pay attention. In the same vein, hospitals want consumers to notice when they receive awards from companies that compile health care data."[30] The problem with that comparison is that *Motor Trend* has built up a brand throughout the years as a respected resource for auto comparisons. This type of respected resource doesn't yet exist in healthcare, at least not universally with consumers. So, for now, it's very difficult for consumers to give value to one award over another, which means it's hard for them to value a hospital brand based on that award.

All of these reasons combine to make award-based marketing less effective than most people think. (By "most people," I'm mainly referring to those without professional marketing expertise.) But that doesn't mean awards or rankings should never be touted. Here are some examples of situations where award-based marketing can be effective:

Internal communications.

All of the above caveats relate to external marketing. But any award or ranking worth its salt should definitely be celebrated internally. Awards and rankings should be evidence that an organization is doing things the right way, and it always helps to reinforce that staff is on the right track with outside recognition.

Everyone else is doing it.

In some cases, if every other hospital in a market is promoting awards and recognition, your hospital may be conspicuous in its absence. As long as the expectation for the promotion is that you're fighting a war of attrition – meaning you're not expecting to win, just not to lose – then sometimes you have to do what you have to do. (This might be considered *purposeful* "Me Too" marketing.)

In a smaller community, where overcoming historical baggage is critical.

While awards-based advertising often gets lost in the shuffle in larger markets, the announcement of an award can help an organization struggling to overcome a historically negative perception in a smaller community. The right award can provide evidence that things have changed since Aunt Millie had a nasty nurse in 1975, and often local media will give big play to such recognition.

If it's a whopper.

If the award is truly significant and differentiating, by all means celebrate it. The Malcolm Baldrige National Quality Award is one example. This is an award that has cache outside of healthcare as well, making it more likely to be valued by the media and consumers. Many in our industry believe another example could be the *U.S. News & World Report* with its hospital rankings. From a perception standpoint, these rankings hold value for consumers simply because of the brand equity of the magazine that issues them. However, their ubiquitousness brings us back to the "throw a rock" theory against using awards and rankings in advertising.

As supporting evidence.

Awards and rankings provide excellent evidence that you're doing something right, and have great value when used as supporting points for other marketing strategies. An award logo at the bottom of an ad, or quality rankings used in an outcomes report, are great examples of how to leverage outside recognition.

In the end, the use of awards and rankings is often driven by organizational leadership – the C-suiters, the board, and top physicians. These folks are proud of the organization's accomplishments, as they should be, and want to share them with the world. As marketers, it's our responsibility to make sure sharing these accomplishments is done in an effective and balanced way. But as is often the case in our world, this is easier said than done.

Overcoming "Me Too" marketing by looking outside healthcare for ideas

A great way to break free from "Me Too" marketing is to stop looking at what other healthcare organizations are doing and start to consider how organizations in other industries connect with their markets. How do consumer products companies develop campaigns? How do they differentiate themselves? How do they build relationships with their customers? What about technology companies? Hotels? Entertainment outlets? Retailers? Spend some time with companies that are recognized for their marketing prowess – Nike, Starbucks, Apple, Amazon – and see what you can learn from them. Of course, there will be messages and tactics that won't translate to healthcare. But there will be many more that can be leveraged to help you build your brand and connect with consumers more effectively.

In the end, no matter where you draw your inspiration, remember that doing what everyone else is doing ("Me Too!") will make it really difficult for your organization to stand out in the mind of old Joe Public.

Habit Four – Whack-a-Mole marketing

For some reason (economic downturn, healthcare reform, planet mis-alignment) we're seeing more and more organizations in reactionary mode when it comes to marketing. Reacting to competitive advertising. Reacting to new awards. Reacting to physician demands. Reacting to drops in volume. Reacting to whatever has popped up this week, today, this morning, NOW.

Impulse-based initiatives have always been part of the healthcare marketing dynamic, of course. Because the industry in general doesn't value marketing as a strategic endeavor, marketing departments are often forced by their organizations to be the hammer in a giant game of Whack-a-Mole, smacking frantically at whatever issue pops up. What is particularly discouraging, however, is that this marketing-by-spasm approach seems to be gripping more and more organizations.

This type of short-term based, reactionary marketing approach leads, at best, to ineffective marketing. At worst, it actually carries a much less obvious and much more damaging side effect. The more reactionary marketing that's carried out, the less time, money and energy there is for marketers to undertake and sustain long-term strategic marketing efforts. This creates a vicious cycle as the issues you're whacking at today were likely caused by a lack of strategic thinking yesterday. For example, if you need to increase general surgery volumes by the end of the quarter, no consumer advertising you can conceive will help that. By not thinking and acting strategically today (because you are constantly consumed with putting out fires), your organization is ensuring you will not have time to address the problems of tomorrow, which then ensures more reactive panic later. And so on.

"Right-side of the menu" marketing

Whack-a-Mole marketing has a close relative that feeds on the same type of sporadic thinking, and shows up in the form of unplanned, untethered marketing efforts. The sponsorship of a local arts event. Purchase of cable or radio time thanks to a special pricing deal from the vendor. Placement on the inside-back cover of the program for the local sports team. A lone billboard touting the hospital brand. We call these and other tactics like them "right-side of the menu" marketing, and they are all-too-common within healthcare.

What exactly is "right-side of the menu" marketing? Check out the menu the next time you pull through the drive-thru at a fast food restaurant. Often, the left-side of the menu is reserved for the value meals – the special offerings where you receive a burger, fries and drink for less than if you ordered the three items separately. On the right-side of the menu, you often have stand-alone items, with side dishes, desserts, drinks, etc. Odds are, if you're ordering from the right-side of the menu, you're paying more for your food than if it were part of a packaged deal.

The same holds true for healthcare marketing. The tactics listed above are frequently stand-alone tactics, belonging to no particular marketing plan or overall strategy. In other words, they're "right-side of the menu" marketing. They often pop up unexpectedly as requests from physicians or administrators, or from vendors with a special opportunity. And just like ordering your burger, fries and soda separately, you're likely paying more money and/or receiving less value with these types of marketing tactics.

Rarely will an individual, isolated marketing tactic bring the same results as it would were it included in an integrated effort. That's the whole point of integrated marketing communications – to leverage multiple and different channels and touchpoints to hit more people, drive higher awareness and compel more action. Integrated efforts also allow for economies of scale (creative/design development, media buys, etc.) which keep your marketing costs lower. You simply don't get as much bang for your buck with a stand-alone marketing tactic.

That doesn't mean you should never entertain a marketing opportunity that presents itself unexpectedly or that wasn't part of your original plan. Having flexibility in your approach and being responsive to your market are important options. But the next time you're faced with an isolated marketing tactic that's not part of your existing marketing plan or doesn't fit neatly into a key strategy, you should stop and ask yourself: what value am I gaining by marketing on the right (wrong) side of the menu?

Habit Five – Focus-group fixation

I've spent a lot of time harping on the idea that many traditional means of research – especially surveys and focus groups – fail to provide true insight into consumer motivations because what people say often doesn't correlate with what they do. One of our favorite sources for this philosophy is Martin Lindstrom, author of the best-seller "Buyology" and consultant to Fortune 500 companies. In a 2010 article in *Time* titled "Neural Advertising: The Sounds We Can't Resist" that focuses on Lindstrom's work, the lead-in helps demonstrate the disconnect between what people say and what they do:

"If you're like most people, you're way too smart for advertising. You flip right past newspaper ads, never click on ads online and leave the room during TV commercials. That, at least, is what we tell ourselves. But what we tell ourselves is hooey. Advertising works, which is why, even in hard economic times, Madison Avenue is a $34 billion–a–year business." [31]

How can this disconnect between listening to what people say and understanding how they actually behave affect our healthcare marketing efforts?

Dental sadists?

A few years back, we worked with a large dental practice that wanted to stand out in the market. In the initial meeting, we discovered management believed their best bet was to promote the expertise of their dentists, a decision based primarily on the results of an annual survey that showed respondents ranked "skill of my dentist" number one from a list of values they thought important when choosing dental care.

Think about that for a minute. Now imagine you're buying a car, and someone asks you to rate the following values based on which are most important to your purchasing decision:

a.　style

b.　gas mileage

c.　reliability

d.　engine size

e.　that it won't catch fire when driving in temperatures above 75 degrees

Given that list, which answer do you think would come out on top? Wouldn't you select "e" because after all, do the others really matter if your car threatens to spontaneously combust when driving in warmer climes?

Yet that same logic applies to the survey question on how customers choose a dentist. We don't know anyone (normal) that thinks, "You know, I like it when my gums bleed, or my dentist wields a drill like a jackhammer." So we think it's pretty safe to say "skill of a dentist" is a given when looking for dental care. But that doesn't mean a dental practice should base its market differentiation on that value. Imagine a car company centering its marketing on the tagline: "The Wren – the car that doesn't catch fire, even in the summer."

Stop asking your customers how to market to them

On one level, this story illustrates a bad survey technique, but more to the point, it supports our contention that when it comes to healthcare marketing, organizations need to stop asking their customers what they think.

To many of you, this will sound sacrilegious. Experts implore: "Listen to your customer, the customer is always right, be customer-driven." But listening to consumers and asking consumers what they think can deliver two very different insights. Turns out it's how you listen that matters. The key is to not listen to what consumers say, but instead to watch what they *do*. That's because research shows what consumers say and what they do has little or no correlation.

Perhaps one of the best resources on this topic is "How Customers Think: Essential Insights into the Mind of the Market" by Harvard Business School professor Gerald Zaltman. Zaltman uses research to show that 95% of what influences a consumer's decisions and preferences lies in the unconscious mind.[32] Because surveys and focus groups only tap the conscious mind, accurate insights into the true preferences of consumers are missed. In fact, consumers are not aware of the hundreds or thousands of factors that influence their decisions and preferences, so simply asking for that information will result in predictable answers (e.g., "I value the skill of my dentist"), but not necessarily the answers that reflect future, or even past, behavior. (Zaltman proposed a deeper "metaphor-based" interview approach to tap into that unconscious thinking.)

In essence, consumers don't really understand why they make most decisions, so asking this question can be fruitless, or worse, misleading. Other books that support the contention that companies gain little from asking customers how they think or act include:

- Buyology: Truth and Lies About Why We Buy (Doubleday; October 21, 2008; $24.95) by Martin Lindstrom.

- Selling the Invisible: A Field Guide to Modern Marketing (Warner Books; March 1997; $22.95) by Harry Beckwith.

- Predictably Irrational: The Hidden Forces that Shape Our Decisions (Harper Collins; 2008; out of print) by Dan Ariely.

The same ol' same ol'

Despite overwhelming evidence that asking consumers what they think or want is misguided, hospitals and health systems still do it, and they do it a lot. They ask what consumers think of their advertising, which heart center they would prefer, and how many beds a new hospital should have. And they use the answers to guide their marketing strategies.

Why does this still occur? For some, it's an opportunity to show they "listen" to their community. (Surveys and focus groups can actually serve this purpose, but just not in gaining a better understanding of what works in the market.) The lack of popular alternatives is another reason – "How else will we know?" (more on that later). But the two most popular reasons are, a) because that's what they've always done, and b) "CYA." Many executives feel that if surveys or focus groups aren't conducted, the sole responsibility for a marketing program's failure will assuredly be laid at their feet.

Redefining how to "listen"

This is not to say consumer surveys and focus groups have no value at all. One of the great applications of surveys, for example, is benchmarking change over a period of time, such as a change in consumer awareness or perception of your organization from one year to the next. (I refer to this again in Chapter 5.) From a *relative* perspective, changes in consumer opinions can be enlightening. The key here is trying to understand why consumers think and act the way they do.

So how does an organization gain understanding of its customers, what they like or how they act? Again, you can listen to your customers, as long as you listen to (watch) their behavior, not their words. (One exception is the metaphor-based interview technique outlined by Zaltman.) Some examples of how to gauge behavior include:

Observe

The practice of ethnography – the social science of observing people in their natural environments – is a powerful tool used by leading organizations like Proctor & Gamble to understand how consumers actually behave in given situations. Observations often provide far more insight into potential problems and possible opportunities than traditional research can.

Prototype

Whenever possible, create a prototype and let your customers actually test the experience, instead of simply asking them how they would respond to it. This could be done with a prototype patient room in a new facility, or a new web-based tool. Combined with observation, you'll learn a lot about how customers might actually respond to your offering in the real world.

Test and adjust

For some marketing activities – advertising or PR, for example – it's nearly impossible to gauge how people will actually act from what they tell you. They don't even know how advertising impacts them, so how can they actually convey that? Whenever possible, test marketing efforts to see how responses vary. Use different creative approaches in different, separate markets to see if one or more drives different behavior, such as attendance at a joint-pain seminar. Or, how changing the hours in a clinic might vary utilization in one community when compared with other office hours in a similar community.

All of the above techniques can work in certain circumstances, but the silver bullet of absolute certainty about what works and what doesn't with your marketing efforts can be elusive. There are interesting explorations into the consumer mind using functional magnetic resonance imaging (fMRI) technology, but even those just answer what a consumer may be thinking, not the more important question of *why*. The best option of course is to measure, analyze, revise, rinse and repeat the process. In the end, you need to trust yourself, your team and your partners – those who have dedicated their careers to understanding marketing and consumer behavior – to provide the best guesses when the unknown prevails. After all, some of this is straight common sense. Running a consumer survey that asks "which is more valuable when choosing your care, your doctor's recommendation or a hospital's advertising?" will provide results that should surprise – or enlighten – no one.

CHAPTER FOUR

Breathing life into zombie brands

From the WeeklyProbe:

Ad kudos of the week: Honesty is the best policy

Transparency is one of the hottest trends in healthcare branding right now. At Neptune Hospital, they've fully embraced transparency with a new advertising campaign titled "We're really trying." The 330-bed hospital has suffered from more than two decades of poor clinical care, awful customer service and horrible mismanagement. In 2002, an orthopedic surgeon performed knee joint replacement surgery on a patient's shoulder. (The same error was repeated in 2004 and again in 2005 before the surgeon retired.) In 2006, the hospital opened a $20 million medical spa called "Facetastic" on land behind the hospital. Unfortunately, the land covered a deteriorating portion of the city's sewer system, and the facility was closed and condemned one year later. The system constantly ranks in the lower percentiles of quality, safety and customer service in national studies. Obviously, it was time for a change.

"We heard about this idea of 'transparency' at a national conference, and we liked the idea of airing all of our dirty laundry," said vice president of marketing Tom Teynah. "Clearly, trying to fix all of this was out of the question. But we thought, hey, let's go with this honesty thing."

The hospital says it's too early to report overall results from the campaign, but anecdotal evidence is already piling up.

"I spoke with my 65-year-old neighbor the other day, right after she waited more than 2 hours to see her primary care physician," said Teynah. "Boy, was she pissed. She said she wished she had seen the advertising earlier, so clearly it's making an impact on people."

"At Neptune Hospital, our customer service ranks in the bottom 10% nationally, wait times are mind-numbing, and, frankly, some of our surgeons are pricks. But we're trying."

Brian Gustafson
CEO, Neptune Hospital

For the past 20 years, Neptune Hospital has earned a reputation for poor service and poor care. Our rankings are dismal, and many in our community refer to us as "the Hospital of Death." But we're trying to make things better. And really, that's all you can ask.

Neptune Hospital - we're really trying.

NEPTUNE

Advertisement featured on WeeklyProbe.com

Zombie brands

As you can tell, I love making up new definitions for marketing change (Whack-a-Mole marketing, right-side-of-the-menu marketing, etc.). Here's another, which is making its debut in this book: Zombie brands. What's a Zombie brand? As we know, zombies are undead, mindless corpses that wander the earth with no other purpose but the relentless pursuit of human flesh. Zombie brands, then, are undead, mindless brands that wander the market with no purpose but the relentless pursuit of meaning and direction. If we want to move healthcare marketing forward, we must put an end to zombie brands.

Say what?

Not following the analogy? Let's start with my favorite definition of brand, from Marty Neumeier's classic Brand Gap:

"A brand is a person's gut feeling about a product, service or company. It's a gut feeling because we're all emotional, intuitive beings, despite our best efforts to be rational. It's a person's gut feeling, because in the end the brand is defined by individuals, not by companies, markets or the so-called general public. Each person creates his or her own version of it. While companies can't control this process, they can influence it by communicating the qualities that make this product different than that product. When enough individuals arrive at the same gut feeling, a company can be said to have a brand. In other words, a brand is not what you say it is. It's what they say it is." [33]

One of the key messages inherent in this definition is that if you're an organization with any presence at all in the market, you have a brand – *whether you like it or not*. Those organizations that understand this concept make brand building a strategic

110

imperative. They strive to ensure their brand perception in the market aligns with the brand they want to and can deliver upon.

Many organizations, however, don't get that the market owns their brand, or misunderstand branding in a way that allows them to think that until *they* address their brand, they have no brand. Some leaders simply don't believe in branding at all. In many cases, leaders believe in branding, but are dedicating no resources to building or guiding it. No matter the reason, if your organization is not trying to direct your brand in a strategic way, your brand is out in the market, wandering aimlessly. It has no guidance. It's not aligned with your desired vision. It's left to fend for itself in an over-saturated and hyper-competitive marketplace. It's a *Zombie* brand. And when it comes to hospitals and health systems, it often feels like the night of the living dead out there.

Night of the living dead brands

In "A Marketer's Guide to Brand Strategy," I describe how to develop a brand strategy, defined as "*a high-level, overarching strategy for leveraging branding as a discipline for meeting long-term organizational goals.*" [34] From my perspective, trying to build a brand without a brand strategy is akin to trying to build a house without an architectural plan.

Unfortunately, it's safe to say that those organizations who are in position to tackle branding at this level are few and far between. A safe estimate might be that between 5 and 10% of healthcare organizations are in a position to embrace branding at its deepest and most powerful level (which means more than 90% of them may be zombie brands – scary). Why such a low percentage?

111

1. Branding isn't understood.

Ask ten people what they mean by "brand," and you'll likely get 10 different answers. In healthcare, you might get 20. Branding is often equated with naming, logos or advertising. These of course play a role in brand building, but as described earlier, a brand is first and foremost what your audiences experience. Without a fundamental understanding and valuing of branding by the top executives, any significant brand building initiative is doomed to fail.

2. Branding isn't a priority.

A consultant friend of mine once told me about an exchange he had with a healthcare CEO as part of a strategic planning engagement. The executive had grown frustrated with the process, saying, "We have too many issues to deal with now. We don't have time for strategic planning." The irony in this statement is amazing and unfortunately, an all-too-common refrain.

Developing long-term strategies like branding will, of course, help ensure greater success in the future, but it's not surprising that hospital and health system leaders have a hard time committing to such efforts in the face of incredible business pressures, such as reform, physician relations, payer negotiations, shrinking reimbursement, rising costs, heated competition, growing levels of uncollectible patient revenue and more. So, while some leaders may understand and even value branding, it's hard for them to consider it a top priority given the multitude of threats and challenges they're facing. This is perhaps the most common reason brand building isn't attempted at a strategic, organization-wide level.

3. Branding is one more program on an over-flowing plate.

Because branding is relatively new as a strategy for healthcare providers, it's coming to the table after many other significant initiatives have been embraced: safety and quality programs, innovation initiatives, customer service initiatives, technology upgrades and the electronic medical record. Leaders often fear adding brand building to the plate, given all the other important programs in progress. Of course, branding shouldn't be seen as an additive effort, but instead should shape how all the other efforts are prioritized and approached. Nonetheless, adding a brand strategy process often is delayed until leadership feels it can clear the decks of other programs they perceive to have more importance.

Reanimating your brand

Given these and other challenges, how should a healthcare marketer go about bringing their organization's brand to life? (Or, back from the dead.) Well, as I mentioned before, a minority of organizations are in a position to actually create an organizational brand strategy. But that doesn't mean you have to abandon the idea of branding. If your organization isn't ready for a true brand strategy, don't give up hope. The key is to understand where your organization stands relative to branding, and how far you can push brand as a strategy given that position. The bad news? Few hospitals or health systems are at the point today where they can experience the full power of branding. The good news? There's still a lot of work that can be done – regardless of the situation.

Level One brand building: Within the marketing department

Brand building at Level One entails applying brand-driving efforts to only those elements that emanate from the marketing department. This would be considered the lowest level of brand building given its limited nature. However, for many (maybe even most) healthcare marketers, it represents the only realistic choice given the organization's situation.

Who should pursue Level One

Level One is for healthcare marketers who believe in branding as an important strategy, but for whatever reason, are unable to enact the strategy beyond the circle of their authority, the marketing department.

When to use Level One

- Leadership doesn't understand or value branding.

- Core elements of care delivery have significant issues (quality, safety, etc.).

- The organization has very recently endured significant change (e.g. a merger) or a high-profile negative event (bad clinical outcome, leadership change, fiscal crisis, restructuring or layoffs, etc.) rendering branding a low priority.

- Budgets and/or staff limit the ability to initiate brand building efforts across the organization as a whole.

- A recent branding effort failed, or left the organization with "branding baggage," forcing the marketing leader to keep a low profile when it comes to branding.

Why pursue Level One brand building?

In essence, putting forth some effort is better than none at all. While efforts in Level One can be limited in their impact, they can make a difference in brand building, and they help lay the groundwork for future, higher level brand building efforts.

Pros of Level One

- As long as you have a marketing department, you can work in Level One.

- You can start at Level One today, and the impact will be immediate.

- This requires incremental resources, which can come from existing marketing budgets.

- It lays the groundwork for future, deeper brand building efforts.

- Brand building efforts at this level will help improve the results of your marketing efforts overall.

Cons of Level One

- The most effective way to build brands is through the experience your organization provides. While marketing communications are part of that experience, core aspects such as clinical quality, service excellence, facilities/environmental experience and more are not affected by Level One.

- Initiatives related to marketing communications at Level One not only have less of an impact, their limited effectiveness has a shorter lifespan.

- Marketers will be limited in their ability to improve the brand at this level, because the elements that typically guide their efforts take place at a higher level. For example, without a brand strategy that has the support of leadership, it may be difficult to identify the top messages for the organization. Or, a key service line facing competitive pressure may need future product development support to build market differentiation. Remember, to tell a good story, you have to *have* a good story.

Level One brand building activities

Brand Research: Begin by measuring the organization's current brand value through consumer surveys, focus groups, interviews, audits, and more. Yes, I downplayed the effectiveness of this type of research in Chapter 3 – remember Focus Group Fixation? But consumer awareness and perception studies can be important stepping stones to measuring the impact of your brand, especially when used to track that impact over time. These efforts help build a case for why deeper and broader branding efforts are needed. Don't forget to monitor social media activity to help paint a picture of current brand perceptions in the community.

Consistent Communications/Messaging: Using marketing communications vehicles with consistent messages goes a long way toward supporting a stronger brand. Of course, determining exactly what those messages should be often leads to the need for deeper brand building work, such as the development of a brand strategy.

Brand Design Development: Often referred to as the "look and feel" of marketing communications, the brand design uses an existing corporate identity (logo, color scheme, etc.) to create a new, updated design applied to all marcom elements.

Web-based Experiences: The organization's website offers one place where marketers can impact the brand experience at a deeper level. Here, any number of tools and tactics, including online assessments, patient communities, online appointment registration, and more, can be used to help deliver a better experience.

Internal Education: Take time to educate key decision-makers in the organization – executives, physicians, service line managers – about the value of branding by sharing articles, papers, or books. Raise the issue of branding and its value in planning sessions or decision-making discussions. Create programming with classes, materials, or more to help teach the value of branding.

Level Two – Cross-functional brand building

Brand building at Level Two represents efforts within specific areas of the organization, outside the marketing department, where the brand experience can be enhanced, or a new experience created. Efforts move beyond just communicating about the experience to changing the experience itself, albeit in limited ways.

Who should pursue Level Two

Those healthcare marketers who are maximizing efforts within the marketing department to build brands and who have opportunities to build brands in specific areas within the organization are ready for Level Two. Your organization still faces some of the challenges highlighted in Level One, such as your leadership not fully embracing branding, for example, that prevent you from taking an organization-wide approach. But for one reason or another, opportunities exist to build a stronger brand in specific circumstances. This could be with a specific facility such as an outpatient surgery center; a service line such as cancer care; a specific service such as mammograms; or even a designated area such as the ED waiting room, or the hospital's main entrance.

When to use Level Two

- If Level One efforts are in full swing, and the team can turn to deeper initiatives.

- If a particular service or facility is facing new or increased competition.

- When a service line or operational director with a passion for improving the brand experience expresses interest in engaging in brand building and is willing to share in the effort and resources required.

Why pursue Level Two brand building?

You are now embarking on the type of work that will have a true and lasting impact on your organization's brand, because you will be impacting how you live the brand.

Pros of Level Two

- You're now affecting how your organization actually lives the brand, so your impact on the brand itself will be much greater.

- Results from initiatives at this level (such as increases in volumes, market share or patient satisfaction) can show the true value of brand building, helping to strengthen the case for a broader branding effort.

- Efforts to improve the brand experience of a product or service inevitably will lead to better marketing results.

- Working in a cross-functional way with other leaders throughout the organization helps demonstrate the true value of the marketing department.

Cons of Level Two

- While moving to match the brand promise to the brand experience in isolated areas, you still face a brand gap at an organizational level.

- This requires applying brand building in the "right place at the right time," such as having a service line director who embraces the value of branding or the patient experience. Sometimes, this can be hard to achieve.

- It often requires funding, typically beyond the level the marketing department can support, requiring investment from a specific area or the organization as a whole.

- It requires staff members or an external partner experienced in product/service development and project management.

- It requires energy, focus and patience to see initiatives through from creative concepting to launch, making them susceptible to organizational pressures, changing priorities, etc.

Level Two brand building activities

Brand Audits: Secret shopping, ethnographic studies, and other techniques not only help assess the brand experience, they also open the marketer's eyes to new ways to enhance that experience.

Brand Gap Analysis: Do a deep dive into a specific service or offering to understand the true experience provided, the potential experience that would lead to patient delight and market differentiation, and what it will take to bridge the two.

Service Innovation: As I've already outlined in Chapter 3, product innovation is the process organizations use to develop new products, or enhance existing products, such as cars or MP3 players. Service innovation is the same process applied toward the development of new or enhanced services or experiences. In healthcare, that could be something as simple as a preventive screening experience or something more complex, such as a maternity experience. The goal is to develop an offering so unique and compelling that it stands apart from other offerings in the market. For true differentiation, try focusing on aspects of the brand experience outside of the clinical offering – for instance, service, access, environment, and engagement.

Level Three – Organization-wide brand building

This of course is the ultimate goal, but it may take work at Levels One and Two before the organization is ready for this level of change. Brand building at Level Three represents the transformation of an organization that has limited and/or inconsistent branding efforts ("Zombie brands") to one that truly becomes brand driven, which is defined as leveraging branding as a top-level, organization-wide strategy to build long-term, competitive differentiation.

Who should pursue Level Three

Healthcare marketers in organizations that are committed to becoming brand-driven are ready for this level. The most important qualification for entering Level Three is having the organization's top leader not only understand and value branding, but champion it. Without this one requirement, healthcare marketers will find it difficult, if not impossible, to succeed in building a truly brand-driven organization.

When to pursue Level Three

- If your organization is generally strong in most key areas (clinical quality, safety, service, etc.) and is looking to move to the next level.

- When the organization's leadership has committed to supporting brand building as a long-term strategy.

Why pursue Level Three?

As noted earlier, branding seeks to manage all possible touchpoints with a consumer to shape how that consumer thinks and feels about a company, product, or service in a given way. By elevating branding to a top strategy that impacts all aspects of the organization, you will be able to maximize the true value of branding.

Pros of Level Three

- The ultimate in branding – becoming a truly brand-driven organization – will lead to greater success for years to come.

Cons of Level Three

- This can take a significant investment in resources and energy.

- It often takes years for a brand strategy to take hold and show significant results.

- If efforts are not continually supported, this can lead to burn-out or a mistrust of future branding efforts.

- It will require leadership to make hard choices, which is often easier said than done.

Level Three brand building activities

Brand Strategy: Any Level Three brand effort requires a brand strategy, defined as a guiding blueprint for how an organization wants to be valued moving forward. It often contains elements such as a brand promise and brand attributes, and provides direction and prioritization for all future brand building efforts. Developing a brand strategy can take three to six months or more, and requires the participation of organizational leaders, but it is an absolute requirement for organizations that wish to become brand-driven.

Brand Staffing and Council: Dedicating positions such as a brand manager (usually a marketer) or a brand champion (should be the CEO or top organizational leader) ensures efforts will be managed in an ongoing and proactive fashion. Likewise, developing a brand council, consisting of leadership, key physicians, and board members, will help guarantee branding is always a top priority for the organization.

Naming/Identity: The name or naming hierarchy of an organization serves primarily in supporting and reflecting the desired brand attributes of an organization. One truism to keep in mind: it's your brand experience that gives a name value, not the other way around. Nonetheless, changing the organization's name (for example, expanding an organization's name to reflect a broader geographic reach) can have a real impact on the perceived brand value, as can reinvigorating an outdated corporate identity or logo.

Brand Building Initiatives: There are many ways to instill branding as a core strategy throughout the organization. An internal brand launch to introduce a brand strategy, working with the human resources department to tie employee performance measurement to brand standards, or building brand "filters" into existing planning streams, are just a few.

Making the world safer

No matter what the situation at your healthcare organization, pursuing branding is an extraordinarily worthwhile goal. The challenge is balancing the dream and desire with the reality. Honestly assess your organization and dive in at the level you feel is most appropriate, and that will afford you the most success. Even if you're at one of the lower levels, your efforts will pave the way for more significant brand building down the road. And no matter what level you address brand building, you're giving your brand direction and energy – meaning one less Zombie brand on the loose!

⚡

The Lord Voldemort
of healthcare marketing

Zombie brands not scary enough? How about branding as Lord Voldemort? Lately, every time I enter into a discussion with hospitals on an upcoming branding initiative, someone expresses an objection to the use of the word "branding" as a descriptor and suggests I find another word to describe what we're doing. The following experiences give us an indication of why this might be the case:

Discussions between a senior marketer and his system peers about branding inevitably result in angst and resistance because of a negative experience the group had with a branding initiative a few years ago.

A VP of marketing knows that key physicians involved in the project didn't really understand the true meaning of branding, so to avoid starting the engagement off with confusion, she thinks it best that we rephrase the title of the process.

Branding has become the "healthcare marketing strategy that shall not be named" – the Lord Voldemort of healthcare marketing. For the uninitiated, Lord Voldemort is a character from the popular Harry Potter series who has wrought such evil on the wizarding world that everyone is frightened to speak his name out loud, lest they unwittingly draw his wrath. Referred to by all as "He who must not be named," the mere sound of the words "Lord Voldemort" causes everyone within earshot to recoil in fear.

On one hand, I understand why those in the scenarios above would prefer to avoid using a loaded word like branding. Why inject confusion, misunderstanding or negativity into an initiative before it even gets off the ground? If rephrasing a marketing process helps bring participants to the table in a positive way (or at the very least allows them to be neutral), then avoiding the word makes sense. On the other hand, eventually, you will need to call a spade a spade. If what you're pursuing is branding, then avoiding the word in an agenda or process title only has temporary benefits. In addition, sidestepping the use of the word branding for an initiative that actually involves branding only gives power to the "dark side" of confusion and misunderstanding. How will we ever move our organizations forward in embracing and valuing branding as a legitimate strategy if we can't move beyond semantics?

In the Harry Potter series, Harry realizes what he's up against and has no fear of calling Lord Voldemort by name, and eventually convinces his friends and followers to overcome their fears and do the same. Depending on your organization and the experiences you've had with branding, you may need to pick your battles. But the sooner you can educate your peers, physicians and leadership about the true definition and value of branding, the less scary the entire process will be.

CHAPTER FIVE:

Measure measure measure

From the WeeklyProbe:

Citing lack of ROI, Evertree Hospital eliminates chaplaincy

Continuing a year-long strategy, Evertree Hospital has eliminated its pastoral care due to lack of Return on Investment, or ROI. Used in many industries as a tool to measure the relative value of a program or initiative (high ROI is desired), the financial instrument is now being applied more frequently throughout the healthcare industry. The move follows other cuts citing the same lack of ROI at the hospital, including the shuttering of the organization's web site, elimination of the marketing department, and demolition of the parking ramp.

"Look, times are tough, and if you can't prove the positive financial impact on this organization, then it's time to go," said Evertree Chief Financial Officer Al Dunlap. "Hey, even God needs to show an ROI."

Dunlap added that additional hospital services and amenities could follow in the same path.

"Our patient rooms are still decorated using a 1972 mauve, and there's talk of updating the decor," he said. "Show me someone who can prove the financial return on a can of paint, and I'll show you a magician."

Evertree Hospital Pastor Bill Gramm was unavailable for comment. The hospital will be auctioning off pews, crosses and other religious artifacts on e-Bay beginning July 1.

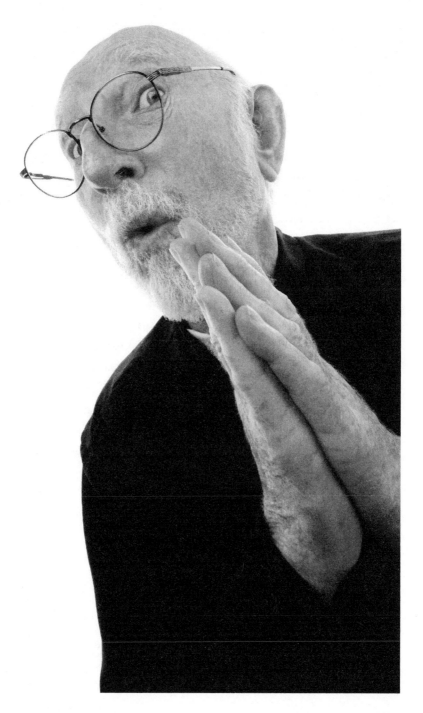

A measurement parable

One day, Marty the healthcare marketer was asked: "Marty, why aren't you measuring your marketing results?"

Marty replied: "I have no clue where to begin. Every time I start to think about it, it overwhelms me. What are our goals? What objectives should we target? Whose approval do I need for those? What are we going to measure? How are we going to measure it? What metrics should we use? Where do we get the data? How will we know if we succeed? I believe in measurement, but I don't really know how to do it, or where to begin. Maybe next quarter."

The following quarter, Marty was asked: "Marty, why aren't you measuring your marketing results?"

Marty replied: "Actually, I can't seem to find the time. There's not enough time to take care of all the meetings, marketing requests, politics, planning, PR responses – my plate is just too full. And my staff is the same way – who would I assign to take on measurement? We can barely find time to meet and properly plan a campaign, let alone build in upfront time to consider goals and objectives. Then there's tracking all the various metrics, reporting, trying to meet to review and analyze the results. Shoot, usually we're halfway through an effort before someone mentions measurement. Maybe we'll start next month."

The next month, Marty was asked: "Marty, why aren't you measuring your marketing results?"

Marty replied: "I could probably figure this out, and find the time and resources to measure effectively, but honestly, no one is really pressing me for it. Sure, we get the occasional question about our strategy, or the 'How do you know this will work?' inquiry from a physician. My CEO wants effective marketing, but so far he hasn't pushed me to validate my approaches, so it's just not a priority. Plus, it's marketing, so people understand when I say this isn't a science. Maybe we don't have to worry about measuring after all."

The next day, there was a knock on Marty's door:

"Hi Marty, I'm Mary, and I'm going to be taking over as the new CEO. Tell me how you determine your marketing budget, why your staff is so large, and how effective your marketing efforts have been over the past couple of years."

And Marty said: "Gulp."

The measurement imperative

This sad little tale helps illustrate what I call the "Measurement Imperative." Despite the obvious benefits of measuring marketing efforts, many healthcare marketers don't make measurement a priority. Given the current climate, however, there may be no higher priority for healthcare marketers today than dedicating ourselves to measuring our marketing results – it is an absolute imperative.

Let me see, how else can I put this?

Please, please, please measure.

It would be my most humble advice that you consider the worthiness of measuring your marketing efforts.

Damn, man, you got to measure!

Who's your measurer, baby?

Measure you must. (To be read in Yoda's voice.)

First prize for measuring is a new Cadillac. Second prize is a set of steak knives. Third prize is you're fired. (To be read in Alec Baldwin's voice.)

For the love of all that is holy... MEASURE YOUR MARKETING EFFORTS.

131

How much do I believe in measurement? If you want to burn the rest of this book and keep pursuing your own marketing philosophies, go for it. Just save this chapter. If you firmly believe that Joe Public cares passionately about your organization and you want to run ads touting your board certified doctors – go for it, just measure. If you love the idea of "Me Too" marketing because your CEO loves it – cool, just measure. If you believe billboards work better than search advertising – that's your right, just measure. To be honest, it doesn't matter whether you agree with anything in this book, and you're finding success in your own ways – that is absolutely 100% fine with me. Just no matter what, you need to be measuring your marketing efforts.

Why is this imperative? Because when it comes to your career in healthcare marketing, measurement is a life or death proposition. Here's how Chris Boyer from Inova Health System puts it:

"There are so many reasons and excuses given for not properly measuring marketing in healthcare. We're so often driven by comfort and familiarity, doing the same thing over and over without questioning why, or is this working. Many marketers don't have the tools they feel they need, or enough experience with measurement or financial terminology, or whatever. But I say, that's fine, don't worry about it. I'm sure your successor will figure it out."

The best defense is a strong offense

Calling marketing measurement a matter of life or death may sound extreme, but from a career perspective, it may not be too far off the mark. As a healthcare marketer, your ability to survive long term in an industry that undervalues and misunderstands your discipline may well rest solely in your ability to demonstrate the impact you have on your organization.

Most marketers do battle every day to defend their budgets, their departments, and sometimes even their positions. Many of you are dealing with business leaders – CEOs, CFOs, key physicians – who often have little or no concept of how marketing truly works or how it benefits the organization. As financial pressure on the healthcare industry continues to mount – primarily a result of dropping reimbursement and tightfisted consumers – the pressure on you to prove the worth of your efforts will also continue to increase. When it comes to justifying the value of your marketing efforts, the best defense will be a strong offense. Meaning: You must begin to drive how marketing success is defined. You must become a master of measuring marketing results.

The ability to drive how success is defined comes from knowing how to track and demonstrate success. As you become more adept at this, your leadership will follow. But consistently measuring marketing results will do more than just allow you to gain the upper ground with leadership. Perhaps the best reason to measure the impact of your marketing efforts is that it is the only true way to know what works and what doesn't, and to continually improve your marketing results over time.

A two-pronged strategy for measuring marketing results

For many healthcare marketers, measuring the effectiveness of their efforts is easier said than done. On the basis of informal surveys and feedback from marketers, it would be safe to say that perhaps 25% of healthcare marketers are measuring their results on a consistent, sophisticated basis. Perhaps another 25% measure here and there, focusing on different methods or using different tools depending on the circumstance. The rest, as many as half of healthcare marketers, rarely or never measure results. That means roughly 75% of our discipline could benefit from measuring the effectiveness of their marketing in a consistent, smart way.

Although the reasons for measuring marketing results are clear enough, healthcare marketers often struggle with where to begin. I provide an in-depth approach in my second book, "A Marketer's Guide to Measuring Results." But for now, here is a simple, two-pronged strategy for measuring marketing results:

1. Measure at a micro level by measuring specific marketing activities.

2. Measure at a macro level by building a marketing performance measurement discipline.

Micro-level measurement: Specific marketing activities

Demonstrating the effectiveness of any specific marketing activity is the foundation of performance measurement. If you're not sure where to begin, start with your top five marketing initiatives (based on budget) for the year. For each, you'll want to track and measure the impact on the organization. Depending on the initiative, there could be dozens of metrics you could use to demonstrate effectiveness:

- Financial metrics, such as revenue or margin gained, or a financial ROI (return on investment) calculation showing how much money the marketing initiative brought to the organization after expenses are considered.

- Behavioral metrics, such as office visits, inpatient volumes, seminar attendees, or website visits. Although these metrics don't show the ultimate result – the financial impact – they do reflect actual actions in the market resulting from your initiative, and they are often important in tying marketing efforts to a correlated financial outcome. For example: "If 100 people attend our joint pain seminar, our experience shows that 10 are likely to end up needing joint pain surgery, which brings roughly $50,000 in contribution margin to the organization."

- Attitudinal metrics. These reflect the opinions of key audiences, such as patients, consumers, and the media. Although these are among the most common metrics used in measuring marketing impact, they pose a challenge in that people's attitudes as expressed in a survey or during a focus group do not necessarily correlate with their actual behavior. (Remember Focus Group Fixation?). Still, these metrics can provide valuable benchmarks for comparing the effectiveness of different marketing efforts over time.

Once you've determined which metrics you want to track (and which ones you can), use a simple spreadsheet to collect the data. Start by listing all of the metrics you're going to track, then log the results. Include any specific objectives you've set (for example, 1,000 new patients over six months) so you can see how your results are tracking against goals.

To help give you perspective on the data, it is very helpful to compare the actual results of your marketing initiative to results from other, or relative, marketing initiatives. For example, "This year our cardiac mailing resulted in 300 inquiries, while last year's mailing resulted in only 200." You should also look for opportunities to benchmark results against baseline periods, when no marketing took place. For example, you might compare surgical volumes over a six-month period when a television advertising campaign ran versus the same six-month period the previous year, when no advertising ran. Both of these comparisons – relative and baseline – help you demonstrate the effectiveness of your marketing when you can't make a direct financial ROI calculation, and they also help you see over time what works and what doesn't.

Macro-level measurement: Building a marketing performance measurement discipline

Your marketing measurement efforts begin by tracking the success of individual initiatives across a number of metrics. But the real value of measurement comes from tracking multiple efforts over a period of years. Without a track record of measured marketing performance, it is very difficult to put your results in perspective.

Let's say your orthopedics campaign resulted in 5,000 unique visits to your website and 200 attendees to your joint pain seminars: Is that good, bad, expected? What led to these results, and what changes in your initiative might have made a key difference? Is it worth spending the same budget again next year if you expect the same results? You'll need a long-term, broad-scope approach to performance measurement to learn what works over time.

When considering building a marketing measurement discipline, think in terms of months and years. You'll need that much time to create stakeholder buy-in and to invest in the systems and technology – such as a CRM (customer relationship management) system or call-center capabilities – that will allow you to fully measure your marketing results. You'll also need time to simply accumulate enough data to make smart decisions based on your measurement results. A two-year time frame is a fair expectation of how long it will take to build and begin to leverage a comprehensive measurement program.

Although you can measure many aspects of a marketing initiative from within your department, it's impossible to build a true measurement discipline without engaging the rest of the organization. Begin by presenting your vision and plan for building a marketing measurement discipline to leadership. You'll need their support when it comes to working with others within the organization who might not prioritize your measurement efforts as highly as you would like. You'll need to work closely with leaders in finance and IT to access the information and systems to allow true financial ROI tracking. You'll also need to work closely with service-line leaders to help define what success means to them, and to negotiate how much of the business results you track can be fairly attributed to your marketing efforts.

Creating a marketing performance discipline at the highest level should be considered an effort in change management, much like launching a new customer service directive or implementing an electronic medical record. And it will take patience, process, and collaboration to pull it off.

In the short term, successful marketing measurement will be achieved by making steady progress rather than by waiting for perfection. Healthcare marketers can start today by measuring some of their current marketing initiatives, while planning for a more comprehensive approach to measurement over time. Along the way, sharing your results with stakeholders will help demonstrate your impact on the organization. This two-pronged strategy should help those who want to stop playing defense when it comes to demonstrating marketing's value and start taking their futures in their own hands.

How to answer the dreaded question

If there's one question health care marketers fear above all others, it might be, "*How do you know...?*"

Typically, the question is posed by a C-suite member, with CFOs leading the pack. And most often, it's used as a cudgel against specific marketing results. For example, a marketer may tout an increase in cardiac volumes thanks to a new marketing campaign, and the CFO will shoot back, "But *how do you know* those patients came in because of your campaign? They could have come in anyway."

This question is frustrating on a number of levels. First, it can be a weapon wielded by the uninformed to play power politics. ("I'm going to keep this marketer in her place – we use facts around here, not conjecture.") Second, it can be maddeningly difficult to rebut. How do you know your marketing effort led to the identified results? There are always myriad variables that might have played a role, making it hard to isolate the true effects of your efforts.

Many questioners know this, and they are counting on the lack of black-and-white answers to dilute the power of your results. Finally, this question drives marketers up a wall because, in the end, it's actually a fair question. If you don't really know the actual impact of your marketing efforts, how do you know whether they are effective?

One of the best ways to defend against these tactics is to establish a control group for whatever marketing tactic you are measuring. Want to know the true effect of holding joint-pain seminars on orthopedic surgery volumes? Compare utilization histories of those attending the seminars to a like group of consumers – same geographic, demographic and clinical profiles – who didn't attend. Or compare those invited to the seminars to a set of consumers who weren't invited. If you can isolate the seminar invitation as the only difference between the two groups, then you can tie any subsequent differences in utilization – and hopefully revenue and contribution margin – to one variable: your marketing.

Keep in mind that control groups aren't always an option. For example, a community hospital would have a hard time isolating one section of town to create a control group when trying to measure the impact of an outdoor campaign. In those cases, you may have to resort to other measurement tactics to glean insights.

Speaking the language of the CFO

Whether it's the "dreaded question" or arguments over contribution margins, if there's one role in the organization that many healthcare marketers find themselves consistently at odds with, it's the chief financial officer. Just consider some of the comments online from marketers responding to a recent NPR story, "Tip: Hospitals Try PSAs Before Spending On Ads,"[35] which featured an interview with James Unland, editor of the Journal of Health Care Finance. Mr. Unland dared question the financial wisdom and effectiveness of hospitals using mass advertising and the sparks started to fly. There were, of course, reasoned responses and questions about Mr. Unland's perspective, but there was also a lot of denial and defensiveness heard from marketers. In a nutshell, "Why should we take marketing advice from a finance guy?"

Well, how about because that finance guy (or gal) is under the gun to defend your organization and keep it viable in the face of increasing financial pressure from reform, lower reimbursement and cost-conscious consumers? To do that effectively, they need, and have been awarded, a ton of power. There's nothing to be gained by fighting it.

Your best bet is to befriend your CFO, and help that person understand the dynamics of marketing, including how it can impact the organization, and how you can track that impact.

First, examine the language you use when discussing marketing with your financial folks. Take a look at one of most clichéd, misused, dangerous terms we marketers toss around – Return on Investment (ROI). What we mean by ROI and what our CFO means by ROI are often very different, and can sow the seeds of misunderstanding and mistrust.

For starters, there is a true finance definition of ROI that we'll leave alone (a ratio related to a company's profitability). Let's just talk about ROI related to marketing. True ROI measurement provides the net financial outcome of a marketing effort. So if you spent $100,000 on a marketing campaign, and you can demonstrate that the campaign brought the organization $500,000 as a result, you have a net outcome of $400,000, or an ROI of 400%.

The key here is that when using ROI as a measurement, you must talk in terms of money. Which means you can't claim to measure ROI in terms of volumes, web visits, seminar attendance, market share, response rates, etc. All of those are valid marketing measurements, and can help build your case for the effectiveness of your marketing. But they are just that – measurements, results, impact. THEY ARE NOT ROI.

If you claim you're going to demonstrate ROI, then announce you've increased web visits by 50%, the response by many CFOs will be "So what? You said you were going to show ROI, so show me the money!" Of course you can't always demonstrate ROI, and showing impact in other ways is perfectly acceptable, but if you promised ROI measurement, you better bring it.

Maybe this sounds overbearing or nit-picky. But if you want to build a bridge to your CFO – the person who in many organizations can have a significant impact on your purse strings – start by understanding their world and their language. Then start speaking it fluently.

Keep your perspective

While measuring your marketing efforts may be a "life or death" proposition for your career, you still need to keep some perspective. Here are four ways to keep the drive to measure from spinning out of control.

Be patient

"Healthcare marketing needs to become less of an art, more of a science" has been a common refrain of mine for a while now. By "science," I'm talking specifically about our ability as marketers to measure the impact of our efforts, using many of the philosophies and techniques scientists use to discover what works best. Following a rigorous, "scientific" approach not only helps marketers determine what does work – and what doesn't – but also helps marketers present and defend their strategies to others in the organization.

Even with a scientific approach, however, there will likely be no absolute answers, at least not in the short term. After all, science itself doesn't always provide absolutes. Take the extinction of the dinosaurs, for which scientists have provided multiple reasons over the centuries. For a more current example, scientists aren't exactly rock-solid in their agreement on what's causing global warming, or even that there is global warming.

141

The point here is not to diminish the role a scientific approach to measurement can have for healthcare marketers, but to release the pressure of finding *the* answer in our measurement efforts. In "The Marketer's Guide to Measuring Results," Larry Daly, director for planning and business development at Covenant HealthCare in Saginaw, Michigan, takes a great perspective on this issue. He talks about the difficulty in using market share as an absolute measure of marketing efficacy, given other variables (such as competitor efforts or physician capacity) that can affect market share.

Daly: *"It helps for everyone to understand that it's an imperfect science. But just because it's sketchy doesn't mean you don't pursue a scientific approach to measurement. To use a clinical metaphor, it may not be as good as a digital thermometer, but it is better than putting your hand on a forehead and saying, 'Seems warm.'"* [36]

It may take years of marketing measurement to feel confident in what works best in a given situation or market. But in the end, even when there may be no 100% absolute answer, the knowledge and improvement gained along the way is well worth the effort. In the meantime, try to establish the right perspective on measurement with leadership and physicians. Consider a common healthcare practice: grand rounds. In grand rounds, physicians review a patient case together, and discuss the actual treatment, the results, and how the case might have been approached differently. This discussion is not held with judgements about right or wrong – it's not a trial seeking to assign blame. It's an atmosphere that encourages open, objective dialogue, and the whole purpose is for participants to learn, so they can apply new ideas and suggestions the next time around.

Presenting the results of your marketing efforts to leadership, operational managers or physicians should have the same straightforward feel as grand rounds. The presentation should communicate the following, in this order: Here was the marketing challenge, here's how we attempted to solve it, here were the results, here's what we've learned, and here's how we might do it differently next time. Encourage questions, suggestions and feedback from non-marketers. This will, first and foremost, establish you as someone who is confident and who wants to master this work. And you're also likely to learn from other attendees, which will help you next time around.

The next time you're presenting results of your marketing campaign, try taking this approach. Even consider raising the example of grand rounds at the outset, and setting expectations for how you would like others to consider the results and contribute to the learning.

Be careful when setting targets

Expectations are a funny thing. A former president famously attributed his political success to setting low expectations and then beating them. While some might argue he struggled to accomplish even that, his point is worth considering when it comes to how you set objectives for your healthcare marketing efforts. It's the old "perception vs. reality" equation at work again – the perception of whether you hit or miss your established target can be more powerful than the actual results themselves.

In many cases, the problem is that without a track record of measurement to guide you in knowing what to expect from a marketing initiative, you're making an undereducated guess. As I note in "A Marketer's Guide to Measuring Results," this can lead to trouble:

"The danger with setting objectives is that once they're articulated, they can often represent success or failure within the organization, regardless of whether they were set with a clear understanding of what is to be expected. If you hope to increase orthopedic volumes 10% with your marketing campaign and you state that as the top objective, there will be some who will consider a 9% increase failure." [37]

And on the other end, aim too low, and leadership may question the value of the effort – "if we only expect to increase volumes 1%, what's the point?"

If you're just beginning to measure your marketing efforts in a consistent way, you may want to consider not assigning a specific target to your marketing initiative. You still should always articulate a goal – "increase volumes" or "improve awareness" – and measure your results. But until you can make a smart guess about what your expected outcomes should be, you may be better off without one at all. Success can be determined by an effort ROI calculation, and if that's not possible, by comparing the results to a baseline period where no marketing occurred.

Don't let the drive for ROI kill new ideas

We covered this in Chapter 2, but it bears repeating. When it comes to healthcare marketing, one of the most frustrating comments from executives, physicians and operational leaders is this: "If you can't prove this will work, then we're not doing it."

Over time, a measurement discipline will allow you to demonstrate marketing's value to leadership, to hopefully "prove" its worth. But when the idea is brand new, it hasn't been done before, either by you and your organization, or (even worse) by anybody else. Of course, launching a new idea before anyone else can lead to great success (iPod, TiVo, Starbuck's "third place," etc.).

But in a conservative culture, the lack of a proven track record is often what kills an innovative idea. The 2010 *Businessweek* article titled "Innovation's Accidental Enemies" written by Roger L. Martin and Jennifer Riel does a great job of reminding us why the lack of a proven track record should be considered an opportunity, not a deficit.

The article leads off with a story of a bank CEO presented with a new approach to finding and landing high-end customers. The CEO asks "Have any other big banks done this?" and the consultant answers, excitedly, "No, you'll be the first!" The CEO then kills the idea on the spot. (Insert rimshot here.) The authors go on to provide a different type of thinking that can help organizations keep an open mind to opportunity called "abductive" thinking. Instead of using inductive or deductive thinking – both of which rely on existing information to make conclusions – abductive thinking is the "logic of what could be." From the article:

"Asking what could be true – and jumping into the unknown – is critical to innovation." [38]

So as you work on your marketing planning, consider the following. Have you left room for innovative ideas? Are you considering trying something you've never tried before, or better yet, what no one has ever tried before? Learning how to use abductive reasoning might help you respond to the inevitable challenge of "prove it."

Don't let measurement overpower common sense

I once met with a frustrated healthcare marketer who told me of her battle with a leadership group that struggled to understand marketing. The strategy in question was a service-line initiative supported in part by, let's say, $50,000 in awareness advertising (the names and numbers have been changed to protect the innocent). After outlining the campaign, the service-line manager turned to the marketing director and said, "So can you guarantee me that if we spend this $50,000 in advertising, it will bring me $100,000 in business?" The inference, of course, was that if you can't demonstrate a financial return, then it must not be a smart strategy.

Here's the problem. ROI is a double-edged sword that can be used to chop down smart strategies and new ideas simply because they're hard, or even impossible, to measure. Frustration sets in because too often, we hear of circumstances where a legitimate marketing initiative is held up or shot down because ROI is wielded as a weapon of mass-marketing destruction. As in the example given above, most healthcare services do not lend themselves to immediate action by a consumer. In many cases, awareness and perception needs to be created to support other aspects of the marketing strategy, all in the hope that more patients will turn to your service if and when they need it. So, for example, it should not be expected that advertising used to promote a hospital's general surgery offering will drive people in to try out gallbladder surgery.

Many important success factors for an organization – brand building, the patient experience, social media adoption, etc. – simply cannot be measured using true financial ROI. But neither can many other components of delivering healthcare. What's the ROI of providing Blackberrys to all your physicians? What's the ROI of repainting your patient rooms in a more friendly tone? What's the ROI of landscaping your facility? Or, as I heard one consultant put it once, "What's the ROI of putting your pants on?"

CONCLUSION:
Future state

On the plane ride back from a recent healthcare marketing conference, I took time to reflect on the fantastic content and discussions I experienced. I heard national speaker David Meerman Scott, who delivered his keynote, "Real-Time Marketing: How to Instantly Engage Your Market and Connect with Customers." When he made the point that organizations need to provide people with compelling content because "nobody cares," I knew he was a man after my own heart. A lot of the conversations at the conference seemed to revolve around the onslaught of emerging strategies and tools available to healthcare marketers – from new social media entrants like Quora and GroupMe to mobile to pay-per-click to interactive portals and assessments. For the first time, it really felt to me that, as an industry, we may be approaching a tipping point where old-school thinking finally gives way to more targeted, more engaging and more effective marketing efforts. Or maybe I'm just a hopeful dreamer. But the key to leveraging all these new toys is to step back from the granular level – How do I build a Twitter following? – and figure out how to strategically apply these tools and techniques. Because no matter what the "cool tool of the day" is today or tomorrow, success will always come from taking a smart, strategic approach to building brand and engaging consumers.

I mention this because while this book may seem like one long rant against the ineffectiveness and silliness I see all around us in healthcare marketing, I actually see light at the end of the tunnel. I see more and more healthcare marketers taking risks, trying new techniques, and at least *thinking* about the right way to build brands and reach audiences. So I'm encouraged, and excited to be part of an industry experiencing a sea-change in philosophy.

To help move us along faster, perhaps we could all take an oath to effect the changes outlined in this book, an oath to move healthcare marketing *forward*.

150

So draw some blood from your palm, join me in a giant hand-holding circle of healthcare marketers, communicators and strategists, and repeat after me:

The Healthcare Marketer's Oath

"I, hospital, health system, physician group or other provider organization marketing, communications or strategy professional, hereby solemnly swear that I will fulfill my duty in advancing my profession by always, or whenever possible, feasible or not career-limiting (and even then, sometimes) support the following changes to how my industry pursues marketing:

- *To orient my marketing efforts around the assumption that Joe Public Doesn't Care About My Hospital, and to help others in my organization achieve the same orientation.*

- *To smash the bonds of the past and embrace new thinking, new strategies, new technologies, new tools and new approaches, and promote innovation every step of the way.*

- *To break the bad habits I or my organization may fall back on time and time again, and to extinguish whenever possible "Little M" marketing, politically driven marketing, "Me Too marketing," "Whack-a-Mole marketing," "Right-Side-of-the-Menu marketing" and "Focus-group Fixation."*

- *To hunt down and transform my organization's Zombie brand, if it so exists, and to build a brand strategy to help leverage our brand to build long-term market differentiation and business success.*

- *To measure, measure, measure, measure, and, once more, measure my marketing efforts, and to leverage those measurements to learn better ways to market, driving greater and greater value to my organization.*

To all of you willing to take this oath, and join in our crusade to change an industry, I say good luck, and godspeed!

To stay on top of trends and conversations related to transforming healthcare marketing, visit ChrisBevolo.com. You'll find a blog, podcasts, papers, other books and more. Drop a note to Chris Bevolo and let him know how you're transforming your organization at chris@thinkinterval.com, or @IntervalChris on Twitter.

ChrisBevolo.com

End Notes

1   Chris Bevolo, *A Marketer's Guide to Brand Strategy: Advanced Techniques for Healthcare Organizations* (Marblehead, MA: HCPro, 2008), 10-11.

2   Thomas Friedman, *The World Is Flat* (New York: Farrar, Straus and Giroux, 2006), 16.

3   "Lowe's workers offered Cleveland Clinic heart care," *Bloomberg Businessweek,* February 17, 2010, http://www.businessweek.com/ap/financialnews/D9DTVOBG3.htm.

4   Timothy W. Martin, "Walgreen to Test Diabetes Services," *WallStreetJournal.com*, January 13, 2010, http://online.wsj.com/article/SB10001424052748704586504574654630471968964.html.

5   Clayton Christensen, "Critical Conversations to Strengthen the Performance of the U.S. Healthcare Sector," keynote presentation, The Master's Forum, Minneapolis, MN., March 5, 2009.

6 Hewitt Associates, 2009 (study no longer available).

7 Henry J. Kaiser Family Foundation, "Kaiser Health Tracking Poll," 2009, http://www.kff.org/kaiserpolls/posr022509pkg.cfm.

8 Sarah Rubenstein, "CVS Shutters 90 Retails Clinics for the Season," *Wall Street Journal Health Blog*, March 10, 2009, http://blogs.wsj.com/health/2009/03/10/cvs-shutters-90-retail-clinics-for-the-season/.

9 Chen May Yee, "Minnesota health care: Condition Critical," *Star Tribune*, February 2, 2009, http://www.startribune.com/business/38730897.html.

10 Nancy Gibbs, "In a Recession, the Consumer is Queen," *Time*, February 19, 2009, http://www.time.com/time/magazine/article/0,9171,1880629,00.html.

11 Chris Bevolo, "The economic crisis: Tipping point for healthcare consumer behavior," *Interval Blog*, March 16, 2009, http://www.thinkinterval.com/2009/03/the-economic-crisis-tipping-point-for-healthcare-consumer-behavior/.

12 Burlington Free Press (article no longer available).

13 Clayton Christensen, Jerome Grossman and Jason Hwang, *The Innovator's Prescription*, (New York: McGraw-Hill, 2009), 90.

14 Al Ries and Jack Trout, "The Positioning Era Cometh," *Advertising Age*, 1972.

15 Marty Neumeier, *Zag: The #1 Strategy of High-Performing Brands*, (Berkeley, CA: New Riders, 2007), 8-9.

16 *By the Numbers,* 3rd ed., (Chicago: Society for Healthcare Strategy & Market Development, 2010), 24, Table 16.

17 Chris Bevolo, *A Marketer's Guide to Brand Strategy: Advanced Techniques for Healthcare Organizations,* 21-22.

18 Brian Halligan, "Inbound Marketing vs. Outbound Marketing," *HubSpot Blog,* July 7, 2010, http://blog.hubspot. com/blog/tabid/6307/bid/2989/Inbound-Marketing-vs-Outbound-Marketing.aspx.

19 Steve Davis, "Dumb Clients? Clueless Agencies? Pick One... Or Both," *Health Care Strategist blog,* July 26, 2010, http:// healthcarestrategist.blogspot.com/2010/07/bad-clients-dumb-agencies-pick-oneor.html.

20 "IAB Internet Advertising Revenue Report," (New York: PricewaterhouseCoopers, LLP, April 2011), 20.

21 *By the Numbers,* 3rd ed., 27, Table 19.

22 J.K. Lloyd, Eruptr LLC data.

23 Ed Bennett, "Hospital Social Network List," *Found in Cache blog,* May 8, 2011, http://ebennett.org/hsnl/.

24 Olga Kharif, "Mary Meeker: Mobile Internet to Surpass PC Web," *Bloomberg Businessweek,* December 16, 2009, http:// www.businessweek.com/the_thread/the_thread_05272011/ techbeat/archives/2009/12/mary_meeker_mob.html.

25 *2011 Healthcare Mobile Survey,* (Cambridge, MA: MedTouch, January 2011), 6.

26 Chris Bevolo, *BrandHope,* (Minneapolis, MN: Interval, 2009), 2.

27 "Hello Ladies: Old Spice's Wildly Successful Ad Model," *NPR,* July 19, 2010, http://www.npr.org/templates/story/story.php?storyId=128626805.

28 Emily Thornton, "Managing Through a Crisis: The New Rules," *Bloomberg Businessweek,* January 8, 2009, http://www.businessweek.com/magazine/content/09_03/b4116030884620.htm.

29 Chris Bevolo, *Competitive Differentiation Through Innovation,* (Minneapolis, MN: GeigerBevolo, 2007), 6.

30 Debbie Kelley, "The Benefits of Making the Grade," gazette.com, April 13, 2008, http://www.gazette.com/articles/benefits-35214-grade-making.html.

31 Jeffrey Kluger, "Neural Advertising: The Sounds We Can't Resist," *Time,* March 1, 2010, http://www.time.com/time/magazine/article/0,9171,1966467,00.html.

32 Gerald Zaltman, *How Customers Think: Essential Insights Into the Mind of the Market,* (Boston: Harvard Business School Press, 2003), 9.

33 Marty Neumeier, *The Brand Gap: How to Bridge the Distance Between Business Strategy and Design,* (Indianapolis: New Riders, 2003), 2-3.

34 Chris Bevolo, *A Marketer's Guide to Brand Strategy: Advanced Techniques for Healthcare Organizations,* 22.

35 "Tip: Hospitals Try PSAs Before Spending On Ads," *NPR*, May 18, 2010, http://www.npr.org/templates/story/story. php?storyId=126899935.

36 Chris Bevolo, *A Marketer's Guide to Measuring Results: Prove the Impact of New Media and Traditional Healthcare Marketing Efforts*, (Marblehead MA, HCPro, 2010), 189.

37 Chris Bevolo, *A Marketer's Guide to Measuring Results: Prove the Impact of New Media and Traditional Healthcare Marketing Efforts*, 92-93.

38 Roger Martin and Jennifer Riel, "Innovation's Accidental Enemies," *Bloomberg Businessweek,* January 14, 2010 http://www.businessweek.com/magazine/content/10_04/ b4164080555772.htm.